FOREWORD

This is a most important history of a most important health pr[oject] timely for two reasons. Firstly, the shocking statistics about h[ealth] and the relationship between poverty and poor health are becom[ing more] and more stark. Secondly, we now have a Government which say[s ...the] relationship and is determined to do something about it. The qu[estion is what] and this history provides some of the answers.

Based on a community development approach with its roots in both the women's movement and Freire, it draws out the connections between health and the conditions in which we live and emphasises the centrality of involving people in decisions about healthcare. These two principles should be the starting point for the Scottish Parliament as Scottish health is given serious parliamentary scrutiny for the first time ever.

These principles have been followed in the Pilton Health Project's many groups and initiatives over the years. The story is totally fascinating, from the liberating approach to mental health in the Tranquilliser Group to the groundbreaking work on health and damp housing to the education through action of the Western General Action Group of which I was privileged to be a member.

Reducing health inequalities means improving the health of the poorest more quickly than the health of the population as a whole. That must involve both improving social conditions and spending health money differently.

Having read this report, and having had first hand experience of the Pilton Community Health Project over the last eight years, I am sure that a national network of community health projects should be an immediate and relatively inexpensive priority of a Scottish Parliament. They would make the connections all over Scotland between health and the conditions in which we live and would help to keep the Scottish Parliament on the right track as it faces its biggest challenge.

Malcolm Chisholm, M.P.

ACKNOWLEDGEMENTS

The work described in this book would not have been possible without the support, energy and active involvement of many, many people. New ideas need champions in powerful places and we were extremely fortunate in having the support of Sir John Crofton, Chair of the 1984 Scottish Health Education Co-ordinating Committee who was the prime mover behind the setting up of the project at a time when community development and health was new in Scotland. His professional support protected the project in its infancy when it was finding its feet and most vulnerable to a certain amount of scepticism from his medical colleagues and his personal support was always there in times of crisis.

I would also like to thank my colleagues, Chista Wynn-Williams, Karen Black and Mary Bain who offered unfailing commitment and good humour during the many years we worked together. The contribution of local people to the activities that were undertaken, not only as enthusiastic participants but as co-workers, management committee members, advisors and friends enriched the project immeasurably – in particular Roberta Blaikie whose active support and wealth of contacts and knowledge of local organisations grounded the project right from its earliest days; Anne Parker and Jean Collie who never lost faith in a dream of a people centred mental health resource; and Marilyn Beagley and Sandra Purnell who kept the campaign for a local minor injury service alive for over five years as well as taking a lead in many other pieces of work.

Thanks are due to Carolyn Maxwell of Lothian Regional Council and to David Pigott of Edinburgh Healthcare NHS Trust who supported and funded the project for much of its life. More formally I would like to acknowledge the role of the Health Services Research Committee at the Scottish Office who grant aided the pilot stage of the project and provided a mini-grant to enable the first outline of this book to be written.

I am extremely grateful to Gerri and Colin Kirkwood, Ian Cooke, Ian Martin, Mike Tait and Lyn Jones who patiently read and commented on sections of this book at different stages in its life.

Lastly, I would like to thank the staff at Community Learning Scotland for their continuing professional support throughout the publishing process.

Jane Jones

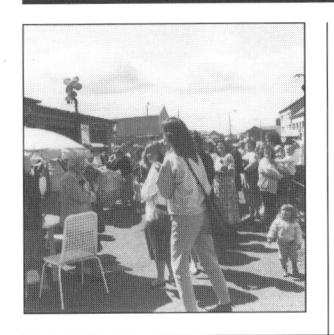

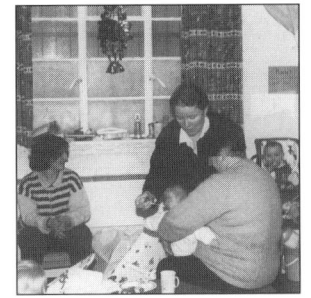

Private Troubles and Public Issues
A Community Development Approach to Health

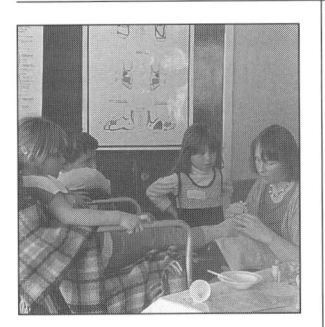

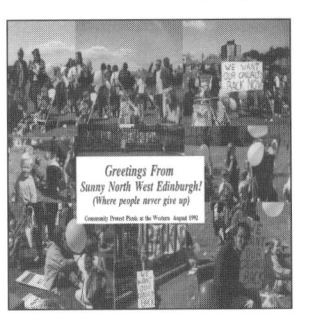

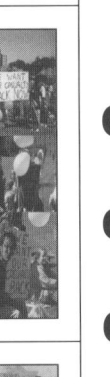

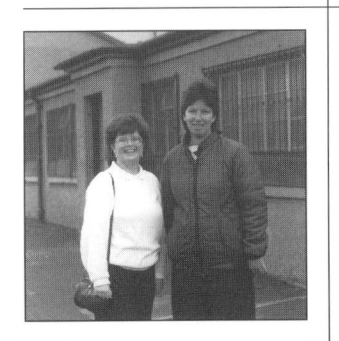

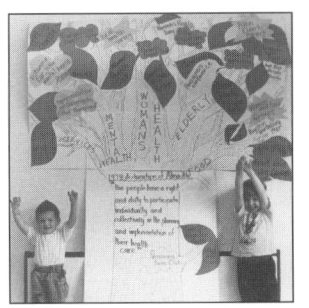

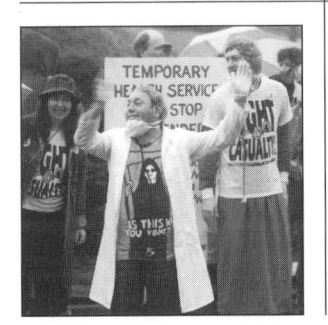

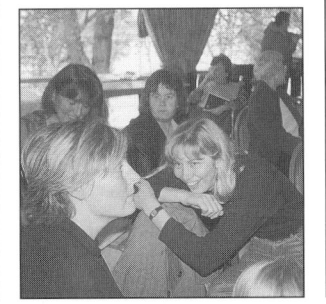

CONTENTS

PAGE

Chapter 1 Introduction   1

Chapter 2 Defining Health   13

Chapter 3 Purpose and Process   29

Chapter 4 Conflict and Co-operation   51

Chapter 5 Community Control   71

Chapter 6 Power and Professionals   83

Chapter 7 We Make the Road by Walking   105

Chapter 8 The Last Word: Local Voices   129

Appendix   157

Introduction

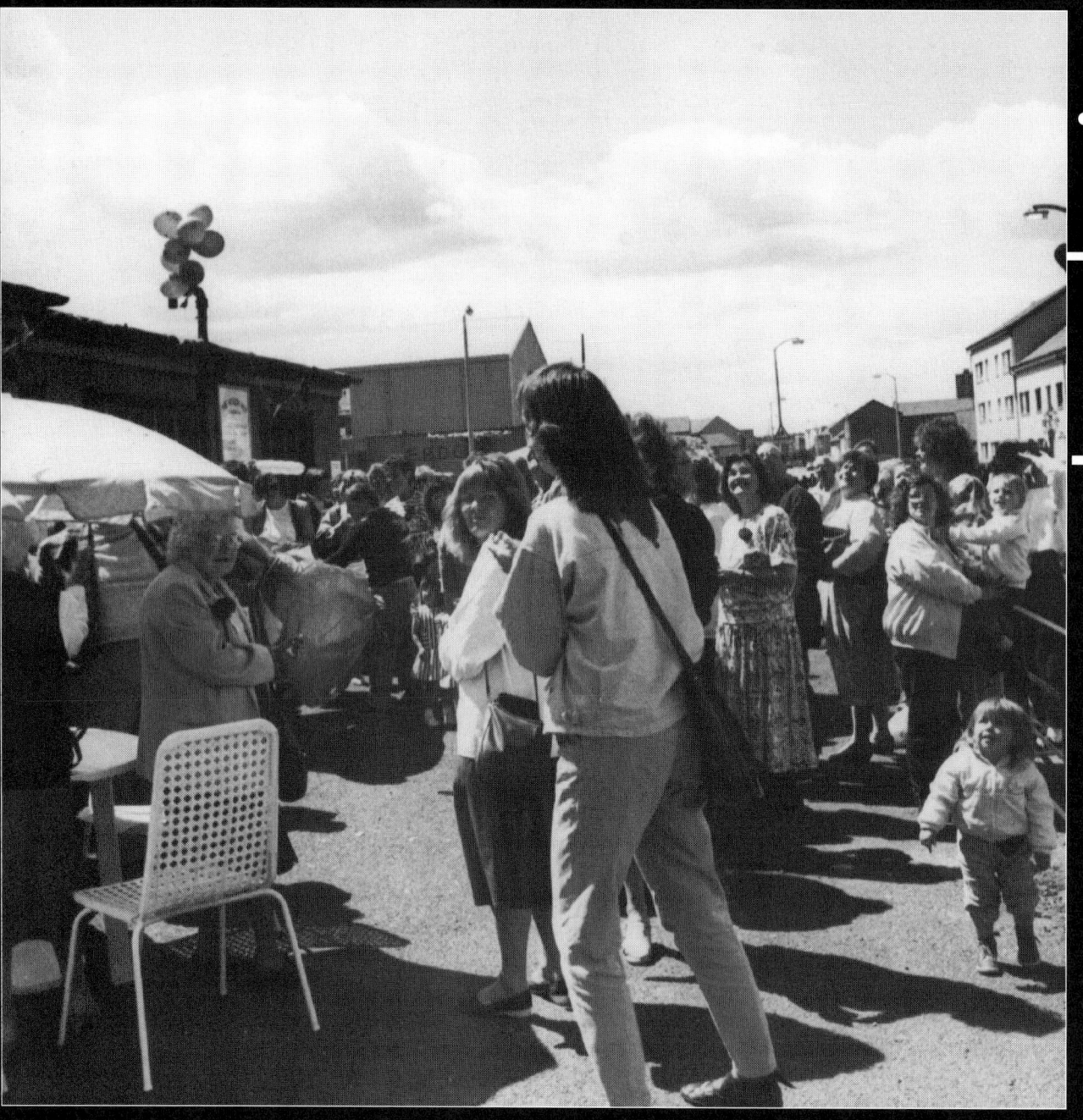

The opening of the Health Hut in 1988.

This book is a reflection on some key aspects of the work of the Pilton Health Project between 1984 and 1994. The project was amongst the first wave of community health initiatives which emerged in the UK as a response to, and part of, the social and political changes that were taking place during the 1970's and early 1980's. Setting the project in an historical context is important in order to understand some of the approaches it adopted and the constraints and opportunities it faced.

The Historical Context

After the NHS had been established in 1948, there had been little disagreement over its founding principles – of providing a universal health service available to all and free at the point of need. Initial queries and challenges over its cost subsided as it became apparent to politicians on all sides that the NHS had tremendous popular support within the country and was one of the most successful pieces of social legislation carried out by the post-war government. This political consensus held for almost 35 years and the NHS appeared to be part of the normal fabric of British life and not open to public debate until the 1970's when a number of social, economic and political changes swept this aside and exposed deeper contradictions and conflicting ideologies.

Firstly, the global economic crisis which erupted in 1974 drove growth into reverse gear and there were calls for a reduction in public expenditure. The first closures of acute hospitals, in London and in the south of England, began shortly afterwards. In Scotland, the higher level of expenditure on the health service per head of population provided a measure of protection for a few years but gradually cuts in the health service were also implemented north of the border.

Secondly, the 1974 re-organisation of the NHS, which had been expected for some time as politicians observed a continuing rise in expenditure, was a reflection of the new ideology of 'efficiency' and rationalisation.

Lastly, there were many different voices expressing a growing concern with health and with health care. The closure of hospitals produced the first anti-cuts campaigns in London which, after an initial concern to simply defend existing services, began to stimulate a wider and more critical discussion about the nature and priorities of the health service. The rapid increase in the unionisation of health workers also allowed new voices to be heard. The strike by NUPE workers in an attempt to close the private wing in Charing Cross Hospital in central London was followed by other sporadic forms of strike action across the country and precipitated the 1974 Labour Party's battle with hospital consultants over pay beds, led by the left wing Minister for Health, Barbara Castle.

The 1974 NHS Act had also created local health councils which although constrained by resources and remit, were active in representing the interests of the public. There were radical developments in public and environmental health and the emergence of 'Politics of Health' groups

CHAPTER 1

around the country which critically analysed the role of the drug industry or the methods of food production in determining the nation's health. This multiplicity of new community based organisations focused around health issues led to a broader debate concerned with the distribution of resources for health, the type of services that were being provided, and the economic and social determinants of health and ill-health.

The women's movement of the late 1960's and early 1970's added a further authoritative force for change within the health arena, a force which had a major influence on the early health projects. One of the key slogans of that movement – 'the personal is the political' – was not only a rallying cry but described the basis for a form of popular education which swept Britain and the USA in the late 1960's and early 1970's. Small groups of women spontaneously formed themselves into consciousness raising groups which de-constructed previous assumptions about gender, re-appraised social relations and became centrally concerned with the role of medicine and women's health.

The women's movement's emphasis on critical consciousness raising as a collective experience, validating personal experience, demystifying medical knowledge and politicising women's health led to an agenda that focused on the definition of health and the ownership of knowledge.

The Women's Liberation movement challenged the way that medicine defined and controlled significant areas of women's lives. Social and personal relations became identified with political activity in which the domestic, and the personal, as well as the structural were acknowledged as significant sites of struggle. Personal and intimate experience was not seen as isolated, individual or undetermined but social, political and systemic.

This challenge to medical dominance over the definition and the analysis of health and illness, and its disproportionate influence over health policy and practice, was not solely undertaken by feminists. During the same period in the early 1970's, it became the focus for a variety of other critics, including academics and polemicists. The role and the power of the profession of medicine and the social construction of illness came under sociological scrutiny in two major works by the

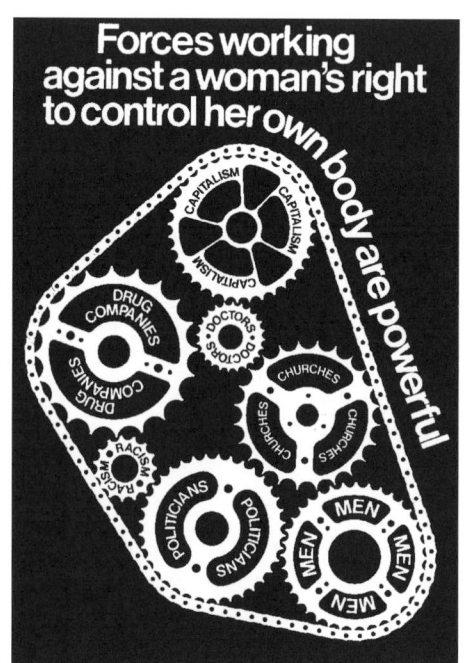

Leaflet from the 1980's National Abortion Campaign.

American sociologist Eliot Freidson (Freidson 1970). Four years later, Thomas McKeown argued that the contribution of medical science in improving health during the nineteenth and early twentieth century had been inflated and that the improvements that had occurred were more to do with food supplies, and improved economic and public health measures (McKeown 1974). Medicine's role as a major institution of social control was analysed (Zola 1972), and the growing influence of medicine over ever larger areas of life – the 'medicalisation' of life was also criticised (Illich 1974).

This current of public opinion in relation to medicine was also to be expressed in wider debates on the international stage during the 1970's. The role of the conventional health sector within the Third World was an important target for the development debate. Studies commissioned by the World Health Organisation (WHO) during this time, documented the shortcomings of conventional medical approaches to health and alternative solutions were suggested, drawn from the socialist development strategies of countries such as Cuba and Tanzania. These principles, which formed the basis of the 1978 Alma Ata Declaration that 'the people have a right and duty to participate individually and collectively in the planning and implementation of their health care', were enthusiastically taken up by a developing community health movement in the UK.

There was a concern with the need to redistribute resources to meet the basic health needs of impoverished people, to integrate health services within a more comprehensive social and economic programme and to see community participation in health planning and implementation as a basic democratic right.

These ideas were carried back to the UK by a number of researchers and community development workers who had returned after working on health development programmes in India, Africa and South America and who provided an influential and radical voice within the field of community development and health work. For example, the work of John Hubley in the West of Scotland in the late 1970's.

The effect of these broadening debates and critiques was not only to create a conceptual framework for a new understanding of the political and social determinants of health but to identify a new role for community work and community development.

Community Development and Health

A community development approach to health began to emerge as a new form of practice in the late 1970's and early 1980's with many of the projects growing directly out of grassroots action. In 1976 a privately funded organisation, the Foundation for Alternatives, influenced by the ideas of Ivan Illich, established six community development health projects around the UK. The majority of the workers in these projects came from a community work background and their remit was to develop community participation and to explore the role of neighbourhood health workers. More projects emerged but initially they were a peripheral activity, largely funded outwith the NHS, through charitable trusts or the urban programme, and seen as either radical, innovatory or quasi-experimental. Their future was uncertain and funding was insecure.

In the late 1970's some of the characteristics of these neighbourhood health projects in London were described as follows:

'They all try to counter the predominant individual and disease-based models of ill-health on which our health services are organised, recognising that ill-health is actually created by society in various ways. Their activities reflect a recognition of the relationship between social class, poverty and health and the inequalities in health provision that exist between deprived and more affluent areas. All of the projects employ workers trained and experienced in community work rather than in medicine, nursing or health education, to work on health issues in small defined geographical areas.

What they are doing is creating a climate in which some of the most oppressed and deprived sections of our urban communities can find a voice to challenge the forces which both determine their health and control the quantity and quality of health services to which they have access.'

(Rosenthal 1983)

Helen Rosenthal, writing about these early developments, drew attention to both the importance of radical education and consciousness raising in this new form of community development work and the inevitable contradictions that this work would produce, in dealing with the health service.

'Attempts by people in the community to address health issues in anything but a voluntary and private way will often be greeted with unease and suspicion by medical and health professionals.'

She also noted, with admirable foresight, that the other reaction to these attempts would be to colonise the initiative and bring it into the safe confines of the Health Service.

However, within Scotland, as in the rest of the UK, health was still an uncharted area for mainstream community work. Many workers felt they lacked the mandate or the knowledge to intervene in an area covered by medical experts or were more concerned with the 'hard' issues of housing or unemployment which fitted the prevailing structural analysis of the time. For example the national Community Development Project (CDP) which operated from 1969 to 1978 and which became for many a model of radical community work, paid little attention to health issues despite the evidence of the link between poverty and ill-health. It focused more exclusively on issues within the public rather than the private sphere (Green and Chapman 1990). An editorial of a report of a conference organised by the West of Scotland branch of the community training group held in Glasgow in 1980, noted that, *'despite overwhelming evidence for the greater ill-health of working class disadvantaged groups, health issues have received little attention from community workers'*

An exception was the excellent Gorbals Anti-Dampness Campaign between 1975-8 (Bryant 1979), and in Renfrewshire in the West of Scotland, where local community workers saw the links between dampness and ill health and supported a local dampness action group. A link was made with this work and John Hubley in Paisley College who wrote a number of papers at the end of the 1970's and early 1980's drawing attention to the need for a link between community education, community development and health education (Hubley 1978). In 1983 health moved up the agenda in Strathclyde Regional Council and they commissioned a review of the potential role of community development in the field of health inequalities (CPF 1983).

Alongside these developments, the publication of the Black Report in 1980 provided evidence of the NHS's failure to reduce increasing inequalities in health and it made the link between poverty, social class and health. The rhetoric of community development, community participation, and community empowerment began to become commonplace in health promotion literature. Health policy documents contained references to increased responsiveness to community needs.

As the NHS tried to absorb a range of policy changes in the late 1980's community development began to be seen from many different and perspectives, as offering some solutions to the welfare crisis. This led to an increased interest in community development and health and a number of initiatives like the Pilton Health Project, were to become funded and supported by health authorities and local authorities.

This second wave of community health workers came from all types of backgrounds – those with community work experience, from teaching, nursing, social work, from activists in the women's movement, self-help groups and political activists. Community development was a term used liberally in the community health field and apart from a few authors such as Wendy Farrant (1991), without much attention to or debate about its colonial history or the

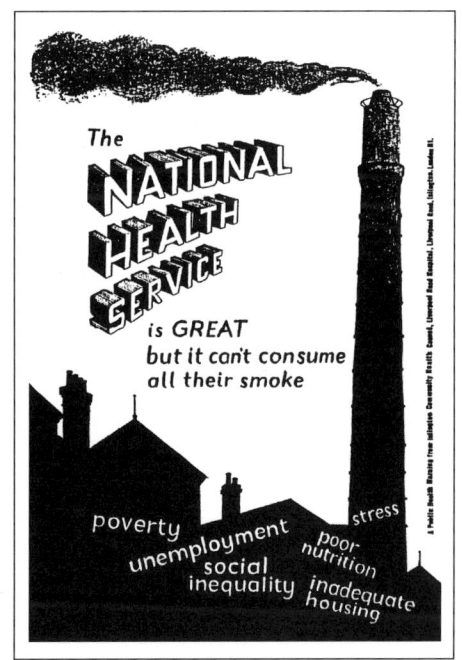

From Radical Community Medicine – a journal of the politics of health 1982.

CHAPTER 1

distinctions between different approaches and definitions of what this meant in practice. This is nothing new and is still continuing. The debates and distinctions between community work, community education, community development, community action, or community organisation are still being elaborated as practice develops in new areas and political structures change. In this sense the Pilton project was simply part of this wider process. We were trying to define what we understood community development and health to mean in practice and to compare this with the broader debates taking place in a changing world.

The Pilton Health Project

In 1984, a report by the Scottish Health Education Co-ordinating Committee (SHECC) entitled 'Health Education in Areas of Multiple Deprivation' noted that the time was ripe to explore possibilities of extending existing or planned community development projects in the direction of health. Following the report, a steering group, initiated by Sir John Crofton and comprising representatives from the local authority, general practitioners, the Health Board, health education, social work and nursing services was established and in 1984 obtained funding from the Scottish Health Education Group and the Scottish Office to establish a pilot action research project. The SHECC report had noted the lack of involvement by GP's in community based health initiatives and the action research phase of the project was subsequently based in a general practice in the Royston/Wardieburn area of Pilton.

Between 1984-1994, the project had three different names and three different homes –within a general practice, within a primary school and lastly within an old clinic building.

Each of the three different locations had an impact on the growth and direction of the project and provided a rich source of experience and learning.

Phase 1: Royston/Wardieburn Health Project 1984-6

From 1984 the project operated as an action research initiative from a base within the Crew Road medical practice with myself as the community development/action research worker. The Royston/Wardieburn area covered by the project in this initial phase contained approximately 1300 households, two local primary schools, a secondary school, two small shopping centres, a community centre and a number of churches.

The whole concept of community development and health was new to the practice and there were many uncertainties and assumptions which had to be worked through. For example, at first the idea of a health project was understandably seen as threatening or presumptuous by professionals such as health visitors who saw themselves as having a longer tradition as community based health workers. Easy access to the project was another initial problem. The accommodation in the practice was a tiny room which had been used as a kitchenette. One of the first tasks was to paint and varnish a wooden top as a desk which replaced the sink. This room was upstairs – an area not usually entered by patients. Initially there was no phone or typewriter. However the limitations of access and accommodation became a positive challenge which forced the work out into the community. Rooms for meetings or groups had to be found from local churches or community centres and community education provided help with minibuses and funds for tutors or crèches. As there was no space for more than two people in the room, the work was more often out in the street and in people's homes.

The limited funding for staff and revenue costs was supplemented by two local agencies. A community worker from the local Pilton Workshop and a home economist from the social work department gave invaluable support and time to the project during its first phase.

The setting for the pilot phase of the project enabled good community networks to be built up but also helped us realise that the different cultures of medicine and community development would best be mediated by employing a health visitor within the project and moving out into a more accessible location.

Phase 2: Granton Health Project 1986-8

After a temporary stay within the local Pilton Workshop, the second home to the project was a large classroom offered by a local primary school, Craigmuir Primary. This school had an excellent relationship with the local community and had gained the confidence and trust of a large number of parents who used the school on a regular basis. The staff were supportive and helpful and invited us to work with the parents or children in any way we wished. The large classroom served as an office, a crèche and a meeting room and brought us into contact with completely different networks. The name of the project was now changed to the Granton Health Project in acknowledgement of the expanded geographical area which the project served. The Scottish Office provided extra funding for the next two years to employ a full time researcher Neil Drummond, the Health Board provided a seconded health visitor post and the new Lothian Regional Council's health committee provided help with a part-time admin worker and with some running costs.

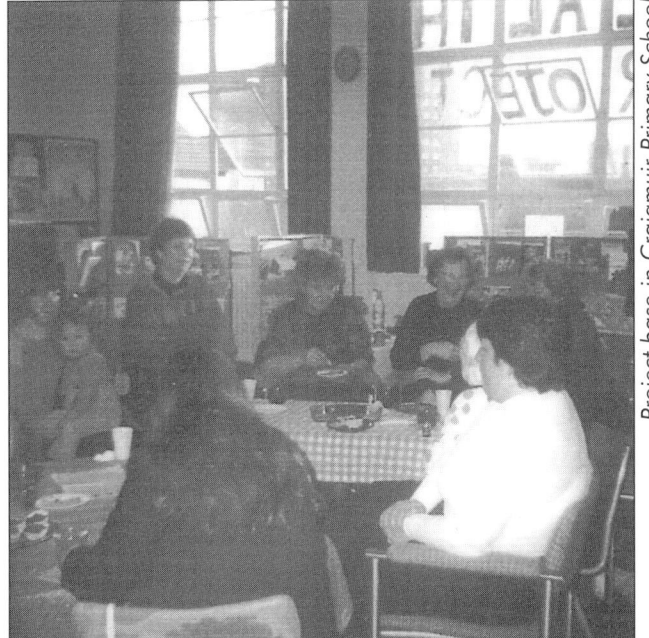

Project base in Craigmuir Primary School

Christa Wynne Williams, the health visitor seconded to the project, had worked previously as a teacher before becoming a nurse and then a midwife and had worked in the local area for many years developing a network of relationships within the primary care team, within the local hospital and in the community. Karen Black, our administrator, was a local parent who had an interest in her community and wanted to become involved in health issues. My own background in social work, community politics, the WEA and campaigning added to this pool of different skills and knowledge which the paid workers all brought to the work.

Local people also brought their experience and knowledge into the project. They became increasingly involved in project activities and in the management of the project so that by 1987, the initial steering group which had nurtured and supported the project through its infancy were able to hand over the reins to an active and committed group of local residents. As the project activities grew, it was apparent that more space was required.

Phase 3: The Pilton Health Project 1998

The last and current home of the health project, known as the 'Health Hut' is an old prefabricated single story building across the road from the primary school, which previously housed the local clinic. The Edinburgh NHS Healthcare Trust supported the project by providing the accommodation which offers a useful variety of different sized rooms. The Scottish Office funding ended after four years and the Lothian Regional Council and the Edinburgh NHS Trust accepted joint funding responsibility. By 1994 the project, now called the Pilton Health Project had developed a number of independent off-shoots, most of which are still running in the late 1990's. The Barrie Grubb Good Food Project runs a fruit and vegetable co-operative from the old clinic reception area and a regular service from its van to local primary schools. The Pilton Elderly Project has an office and a base from which it runs a transport service, and an information and befriending service. A Counselling Service operates from a small counselling room in the project and the Pilton Reach Out Project which outgrew the space in the Health Hut, operates from a purpose built building next door. Apart from the counselling service, these projects employ a large number of local people and are managed by local people themselves. In 1989 Mary Bain became our new administrator, counselling service receptionist, sometimes crèche support worker, typist, general organiser and calm welcomer to the increasing number of people who came to use the Health Hut.

Developing the Practice

As the first community development and health project in Scotland, work was being developed in relatively uncharted waters. Like many other health projects which followed in the 1980's, there was no blue print to follow. As workers, we had a mixed bag of skills and experience but these had to be adapted to the particular setting. For example, health visiting contacts were

CHAPTER 1

invaluable in helping us make links with a network of people who had been individual clients or patients and who might not have had much involvement in community groups or activities but the relationships we were trying to forge were not the individual patient/expert mode but a more collective, equal expert one. Community work and campaigning skills were crucial but had been largely confined to work with people who were reasonably well. Working with the 'imperative of need' with people who experienced depression or more severe illness had to be more sensitive and develop a different pace and approach. The move from individual support and help, to a more collective and political perspective was more difficult and longer term. Knowledge about the health service from a professional perspective had to be redrawn from a community perspective.

The push during the first years to concentrate on developing the practice, was in part the consequence of being under the spotlight, of having to 'show' what the work meant in concrete terms, to handle scepticism in some quarters, of very short term funding (6 months initially) and of being a single worker project until 1986.

The initial location of the project in a general practice also brought us face to face with the realities of developing this new form of practice within a medical setting with its own set of assumptions and values. There was an unresolved tension between working on issues that the local community had identified as important and those which health professionals felt were paramount.

The development of any more rigorous, theoretical analysis of practice took a back seat until much later on in the project's life but from the start there was a clear attempt to declare the particular values which underpinned the work in order to reject the growing move to see problems of health inequality as solely a matter of individual 'lifestyles'. These views which were encouraged by the Tory government and many health authorities were based on the 'social pathology' or 'victim blaming' approach which assumes that health problems were the result of individuals' poor and inadequate behaviour or something essentially pathological about the area itself.

In publicity and information about the project three core values were explained, in answer to

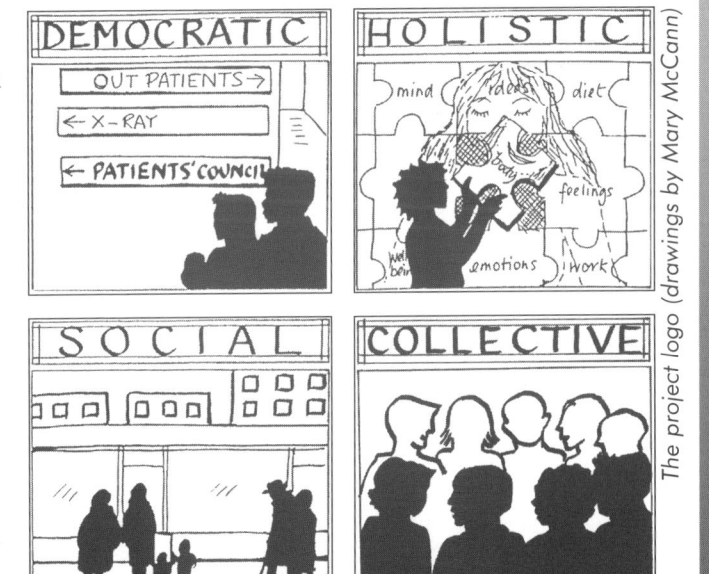

Pilton Community Health Project

The project logo (drawings by Mary McCann)

the question – what kind of values underpin the work? The following is an extract from our first publicity leaflet:–

1. We are working with a social rather than a medical model of health

So we believe that health is as much affected by damp housing or unemployment as diet or exercise. This means, for example, that although we would agree that diet affects a person's health, we would also think that proximity to good shops, cost, advertising and government subsidies were also important. We might also want to explore people's feelings about food and what it represents to them.

This broader view of health requires collaborative working between various professional groups and local people, not just traditional health workers.

2. We use a collective rather than an individual approach

Although we are concerned to help people individually, we believe this is best done by them joining with others to address the problem. For example, someone might feel that they are having great difficulty withdrawing from tranquillisers, they might be experiencing a variety of strange feelings and become more and more isolated. By joining with others experiencing the same difficulty people gain mutual support, reduce their isolation and begin to see common threads in their experience.

3. We want to support a more democratic approach to health issues

This means that we would not only wish for more consultation between the health service and the public but that people should be involved more actively in their personal health care and in the decision making processes of the Health Board.

These values are not just our own. They are values underpinning reports from the World Health Organisation, of which the UK is a signatory. For example in 1978, the Declaration of Alma Ata was that *'people have the right and duty to participate individually and collectively in the planning and implementation of their health care.'*

The choice of work that developed in relation to these values was a concrete way of demonstrating that community health work was a broad based political, social and educational activity.

The chapters that follow try and document some of the practice which developed and re-examine a number of recurrent themes which echoed through the years. Each community and each group of workers will have different constraints and strengths and this account is not presented as a definitive model of community development and health practice but as a descriptive and reflective account of one particular project which had the good fortune to have continuous funding and a relatively stable staff team for over ten years.

References

Bryant, R (1979)	The Dampness Monster: A report of the Gorbals Anti-Dampness Campaign. Scottish Council of Social Service
Community Development Foundation (1983)	Community Development and Health Issues: A review of existing theory and practice
Farrant, W (1991)	Addressing the Contradictions: Health Promotion and Community Health Action in the United Kingdom, International Journal of Health Services, Vol.21 No.3, pp 423-30
Freidson, E (1970)	The Profession of Medicine: A study of the Sociology of Applied Knowledge. Dodd Mead, New York
Green, J and Chapman, A (1990)	The Lessons of the Community Development Project for Community Development Today in Roots and Branches Papers from the OU/HEA 1990 Winter School on Community Development and Health
Hubley, J (1978)	Community Education: Community Development and Health Education. Community Education
Illich, I (197)	Medical Nemesis. Calder & Boyars, London
McKeown, T (1976)	The Role of Medicine: Dream, Mirage or Nemesis. Nuffield provincial Hospitals Trust, London
Rosenthal, H (1983)	Neighbourhood Health projects – Some new approaches to Health and Community Work in parts of the UK, Community Development Journal, Vol.18 No.2, pp 120-31
Scottish Health Education Co-ordinating Committee (S.H.E.C.C.) 1984	Health Education in Areas of Multiple Deprivation
Zola, I K (1975)	In the name of health and illness, Soc. Sci. Med., 9, pp 83-7

Defining Health

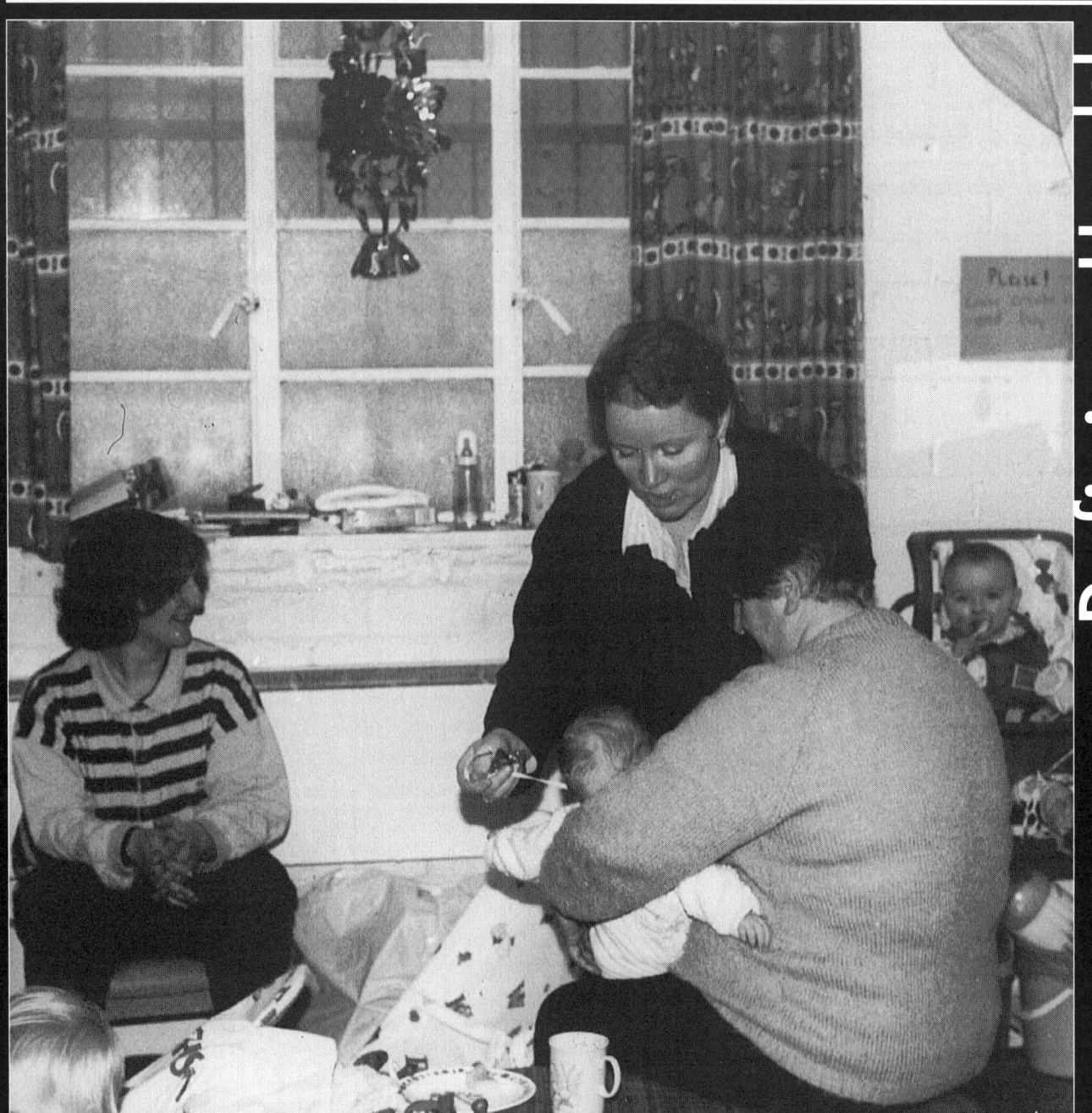

The project's creche.

Introduction

'contemporary public health is as much about facilitating a process whereby communities use their voice to define and make their health concerns known as it is about providing prevention and treatment.'

(Minkler 1997)

One of the core features in a community development and health strategy is to encourage people to identify their own health concerns and the issues that they feel are important. At first sight this might not appear to be such a difficult task. A superficial interpretation might assume that all that is required is to simply go and ask them. Our early work in the health project was indeed about asking people what they thought were the main obstacles to their health and what could be done about them. However the parallel process that was occurring during these informal discussions, was the equally important business of getting to know each other – of building up relationships within which a more equal dialogue could take place. How much could we be trusted? How did we react to what they said? Would anything happen as a result of our conversation? We began to realise that both the context and the relationship within which such discussions take place have an enormous influence on what is talked about – on what is expressed or brought forward into the public domain.

One of the first tasks of the action research phase of the project was to undertake a small local study of the way people understood and perceived their own health and that of the local community. Through this, it was apparent that people talked about health according to how questions were framed, whether in questionnaires or in conversation, and according to how much exposure they had had to 'official' accounts.

During the early phases of the project when making ourselves known to different groups, we observed how people reacted to the idea of 'a health worker'. At a first meeting with a group of mothers in a local primary school we were greeted with remarks such as – put out your fags everyone and – don't look at what we're cooking today, it's probably not good for us! Although this was said with a sense of humour, there was also an undercurrent of guilt. This conveyed a sense that we had 'caught them out' – almost like children expecting to be chastised. This was an unpleasant role to be cast in. We found it frustrating that people had been made to feel that way and that it somehow created a particular set of expectations and relationships. We had to make strenuous efforts to reassure people that we were not there to tell them what to do or what to eat or how to live. The expectations and assumptions behind their reactions explained something of their previous experience of health workers, the health messages being promoted, the relationships involved and the type of communication which may have taken place.

CHAPTER 2

We became sensitive to how people had internalised victim-blaming messages. They had come to believe it was their own fault that they didn't have a 'healthy' diet or that they had suffered a heart attack.

Working through the latter end of the 1980's, within the developing ethos of the market economy, we became increasingly aware of the extent to which the meaning of health was changing, and the effect this was having on the nature of health discourse within the community. Government policy, health education, the media and commercial interests combined to bring attention to individualism and 'lifestyles'. Eating well, exercising regularly, dealing with individual stress, making the right 'healthy choices' dominated discussions about health.

'although there do exist voices of dissent, health professionals, policy makers and politicians have largely succeeded in promoting the view that individual behaviour is both the prime cause of ill health and a major factor in the maintenance and attainment of good health. This view has been reinforced by the media and has entered the domain of "public facts" with very little critical debate about its scientific basis.'

(R.U.H.B.C. 1989)

In relation to the NHS, patients, citizens, the 'public' and the 'community' became re-cast as individual consumers and service customers and invited to exercise their individual rights. However this new 'freedom' only allowed these rights to be exercised in pre-defined ways and through prescribed channels. For example commenting on specific aspects of services such as waiting times in out-patient departments or making individual complaints. These individual comments were then dealt with by the new managers of publicly unaccountable trusts. Local health councils, previously seen as the public watchdogs of the NHS were slimmed down and even more tightly controlled by Health Boards. These structural changes supported the dominant market ethos in relation to public services and the ideological position of the New Right.

Debates about the impact of poverty, unemployment, industrial pollution, structured inequalities, the drug industry or poor housing on peoples' health were marginalised as these major changes in the health service structure absorbed the attention of the media, polemicists, academics and critics. There was little focus on the causes or the determinants of ill-health and this changing discourse was played out in front of our eyes at local level, influencing the way that people talked about health, influencing the very meaning of it.

As we developed closer relationships with people, particularly when working on issues relating to emotional distress or mental health, it was apparent that longstanding struggles for definition were taking place. People experiencing mental health problems drew on many different conceptual frameworks and levels of meaning in order to make sense of their own inner world. This process was more private but when an opportunity could be created for this to be shared collectively, the sharpness of the contradictions people experienced and the clarity of their observations struck us forcibly and also presented an implicit challenge to the traditional bio-medical definition of much mental illness.

These experiences led us to be clearer about the importance of people taking time to define their own health issues. This had to be a part of any strategy which was trying to encourage people to understand more thoroughly the determinants of ill-health, to gain more control over their own lives and to influence the way that the health service they were paying for, redressed inequalities and acted effectively.

Two views relating to health dominated the conceptual context within which we were working. Firstly there was the bio-medical model of health and its association with dysfunction and disease, with a sense of the body as machine, with expert knowledge, with power and authority. Secondly, there was the behavioural change model within health education which sees health as an individual responsibility, defining some behaviours as health enhancing and others as bad and risky. People are assumed to act 'unhealthily' because they are ignorant and will therefore change their behaviour when given the correct information.

These two dominant views influenced our work in a number of ways. People with long experience of powerlessness are likely to have had their problems defined for them by others – on the receiving end of advice from a string of professionals. They are used to articulating what they think professionals want to hear. In the end they often believe this dominant view as 'the only truth'.

Much of our work was to try to clear a space in this web of powerful ideologies where people could explore and articulate their own ideas and experiences in the company of others. A collective understanding and analysis of problems and issues could then be constructed so that people could decide on an appropriate course of action.

The following examples each illustrate a particular aspect of defining health. They show the complexity involved in this process and the relevance of this for the role of the worker.

1. Differing Definitions of Health

Local Interviews
One of the objectives of the action research stage of the project was to assess the health concerns of both local professionals and the local community. In 1984/5 in-depth interviews were undertaken with 18 local residents drawn from a random sample and 22 local professionals, representing a range of local statutory and voluntary agencies. This was when the project was new to the area and the survey was used as a way to engage with people in the community and as a type of 'mapping' exercise to gain an impression of people's views and concerns and to understand how they defined health.

The study gave us our first impression of the complex ways people think about their health and the different perceptions held by different groups of people.

Defining Health in General Terms

In response to a general question about how they defined health, for example, local professionals almost all responded in a similar way. They tended to define health in broader, more abstract terms, using the World Health Organisation's definition of health incorporating a notion of physical, mental and social well-being which was prominent in the early 1980's. We noted how some people struggled to get the words in the right order as though they were being tested. As professionals they had a role in stating the 'official view'. Local residents also expressed this broad perception of health but they drew more readily on their own experience and understanding of what part health played in their own and their families and friends lives. They tended to define health in more specific, concrete and personal terms. For example, feelings and emotions, feelings 'inside' were seen to be important, closely followed by happiness/ enjoyment, energy/alertness and mobility.

This study was a fairly limited exercise, involving small numbers of people but its findings are consistent with other research in this area. For example a large scale national study undertaken by Blaxter in 1990 which analysed people's attitudes and beliefs about health identified four main groups of beliefs that we identified in our own study. These were:

- **health seen as never ill, no disease**
- **health as physical fitness/energy/vitality**
- **health as a state of psycho-social wellbeing including feelings of happiness/confidence**
- **health as a function – being well enough to do things.**

It also supported the conclusion which we drew from our own survey – that health was not seen by local people as a unitary concept but was more complex and multi-dimensional (Blaxter 1990).

Functional Fitness

The way of describing health in a functional context – as 'well-enough to do things' was common to both professionals and local residents in our study. A health visitor commented, *"if people can manage to get out and about, they are doing well"*. An elderly local resident said, *"as long as I can get out for a drink on a Friday and get my messages, I'm doing not bad"*. This category of functional fitness is a theme which recurs in most major studies, and can be interpreted according to different ideological beliefs. Kelman (1975) for example, saw it being entrenched within a capitalist mode of production – as fitness to provide labour for capital. Blaxter (1983) found working class respondents defining health as fitness for 'normal' roles. Cornwell (1984) also identified the connection between 'normal roles', gender and the sexual division of labour in that women associated feeling healthy with being well enough to carry out their domestic and childcare role, men with being fit enough for work outside the home. This sense of health as enabling you to carry out your ascribed role was also captured by one of the interviews conducted in the health project by the Open University who were using the project as a case study for their course 'Health and Wellbeing' (Open University, 1992). This was with a local woman, who had become involved in one of the groups in the project.

'If you're healthy enough to get up in the morning to do what you've got to do without having to worry about being exhausted or breaking down by dinner time. You're happy, everybody's happy. That's my idea of health. Oh yes, no just stop smoking, stop drinking – I do them all but health starts for me – I've got to be healthy for my family. To get up in the morning and do what I've got to do and still have a smile on my face at 10 o'clock at night. To me that's healthy.'

The way that women would often put their own health last, giving their main priority to looking after their children or family also became more and more apparent as we worked with different groups of women. The information from the study helped us in deciding to create opportunities for some protected time for women, with childcare, so that they might have the space to think about their own health. This was highly valued. Work with older women in a middle years group, with younger women with children in a 'Family Matters' group, and planning women's health days with local women, for example, created an opportunity for them to reappraise their role and begin to find time for themselves as individuals.

Different Perceptions

The study also gave an indication of differences in perception about health and about the determinants of health. These differences were not only between local residents and professionals but between different groups of professionals. There were also different ideas as to what they thought determined a healthy community. For example there was a measure of agreement in defining social and economic factors and the need for social cohesiveness as affecting the health of the local area. However, health professionals were slightly more inclined to draw from an individual model of self-sufficiency and responsibility.

'people to be more self-sufficient, very little requirement from health professionals'

'a community willing to accept a bit of responsibility'

'educated about health, not dependent on professionals'.

These differences in perception affected the level of support given by health professionals to the different activities within the project and were noted in the project report at the end of the pilot phase.

CHAPTER 2

'Whose definition of "health" do we use? GP's are more familiar with overall trends in mortality and morbidity and many would see their role in health promotion as encouraging a reduction in smoking or adopting preventative measures such as screening for coronary heart disease or hypertension. Local residents may indeed act on advice or take up screening facilities if offered but sometimes there can be a clash of perspective if local people feel there are more immediate issues affecting their health. These might be things such as housing, financial worries, dependency on tranquillisers or anxiety.'

(Project Report 1986)

2. Official Accounts of Health

Because of the differing perceptions of health, our first task when meeting new groups in the community was to clarify what we meant by health and what we understood by 'health issues'. The interaction described below was not an isolated incident and it serves to demonstrate the way language and meaning, definition and power come together.

High Flats Group

At a first meeting with a group of tenants of a high rise block discussion ranged over many of the problems they faced. Particular attention was given to the faulty intercom system and broken lifts, which prevented people gaining easy access to the block. As well as problems of maintenance and lack of play space for children they catalogued a number of difficulties such as doctors and health visitors not willing to come to the flats, or finding it hard to get in, the high level of tranquillisers being taken because of the stress of break-ins and lack of security, and of people not being accepted onto some doctors' lists from this particular address. When it was observed that a lot of health issues had been identified which we could perhaps look at together, one tenant thought for a moment and looked slightly puzzled and then said 'What do you mean – do you mean about my smoking?' Although she had just described her day to day reality which meant her access to health care was extremely difficult, her children were not able to get immunised easily, she had been given sleeping pills and tranquillisers to cope with the stress of living there, she was unsure that these elements of her experience would be included in the word health. Health – that was about smoking wasn't it?

This example shows the different meanings given to health influencing communication on two levels. Firstly there seems to be an attempt to reflect the 'official' view of health – that it is about lifestyle and behaviour such as smoking – and secondly there is also some confusion as to whether the meaning of the word 'health' includes social aspects such as the impact of poor housing and access to services. This was a first meeting with the tenants and we were unfamiliar to each other. Their assumptions about what community health workers might think had not yet been tested out and I was still very much an 'outsider' to their everyday lives.

The impact of social relations on the way people define health has been well documented by Jocelyn Cornwell in her research with families in London's East End. She noted the different accounts people gave about health in different circumstances. The differences appeared not only to relate to who they were talking to but were a consequence of the particular social relationship involved. She describes these differences as 'private' and 'public' accounts (Cornwall 1984).

She observed that 'public accounts' arose when people were asked by an interviewer to talk about health in general and abstract terms, whereas 'private accounts' were formed directly from personal experience and from the thoughts and feelings accompanying them. In conducting the interviews, Cornwell also noted the subtle difference which led to a more private account being related. This was usually determined by who was in control of the conversation. When the interviewee was describing an experience or telling a story, he or she was more in control of the relationship than when answering set questions from the researcher. In this situation a less self conscious and more private account would ensue. This would be less deferential, contain people's own ideas and would sometimes be more critical of their health care or their treatment by particular health professionals. The power relationship between them determined the way health was defined. She goes on to say,

'our culture assumes that health is a subject for experts, something only doctors really know about, and this has a profound effect on the relationship "ordinary" people, people who are not medically qualified, have with it. The effect was...in their public accounts of health related matters, people made sure that what they said was not only non-controversial, and thus likely to be acceptable, but that it conformed with their notion of the 'medical point of view'... It is always possible to characterise public accounts in terms of their overriding preoccupation with questions of acceptability and legitimacy'.

Cornwell (1984)

The close social and extended family networks of the London East End families interviewed in the Cornwell study must have provided a supportive web of similar private accounts, re-enforcing and creating an alternative legitimacy to the official view. In another study where the research was conducted in groups, rather than through individual interviews the researchers noted that the public accounts in these groups were similar to the more private accounts recorded by Cornwell. It appeared as though the group situation helped to legitimise these private accounts, making them generally more acceptable and in so doing, produce a new public account (Stimson and Webb 1975).

In communities where residents are more isolated and fragmented, through industrial re-location, employment and housing policies, this alternative legitimacy may well be weaker and the public or official account seen as 'the only truth'. Individuals in this situation who feel that their own reality is different from the official view can experience an increased sense of powerlessness and isolation. This has particular relevance in relation to mental health where the associated stigma attached to sufferers, precludes them from talking about their experiences more openly or in the wider community.

Official accounts may well have their own validity but if their dominance obstructs other equally valid accounts from being heard, or even expressed, this not only limits any collective understanding of the broader issues but limits the means of tackling them.

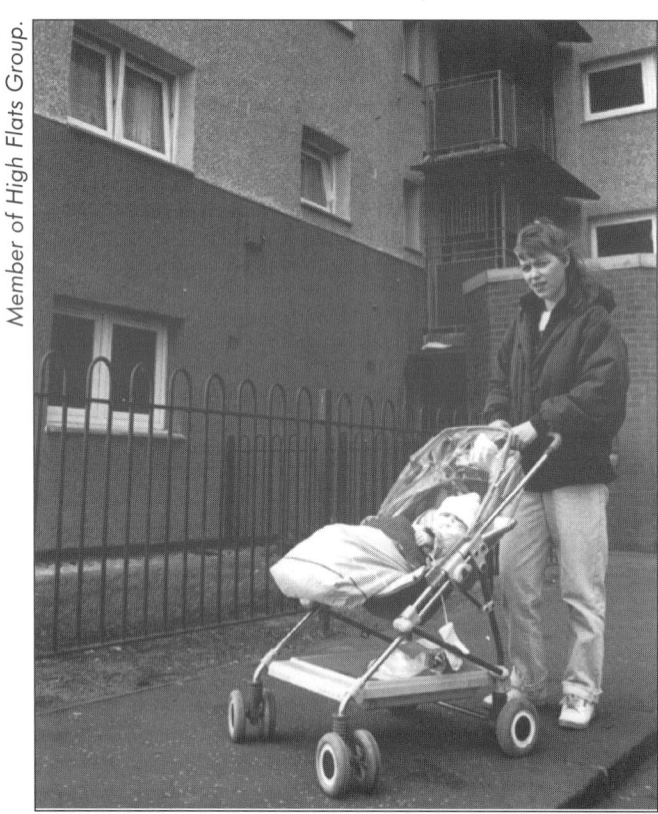

Member of High Flats Group.

Implications for Practice

This task of encouraging private accounts of health to be seen as valid and to be discussed more openly was central to the work of the Pilton project in the early stages.

'People have a lot of knowledge about their own health and what influences it but these perceptions have become less valid as medical expertise has become more sophisticated. Jargon and professional distance can serve to discourage dialogue between lay people and health professionals so that a person's own experience and ideas about their health can be felt as less important. Meeting and talking in informal groups can help people regain confidence in expressing a personal view'

(Project Report 1988)

The act of working alongside people and encouraging them to identify their own definition of the problem or to express their own views about health demonstrates a clear educational role for the worker. This is particularly important when the dominant 'discourse' serves to exclude or discount alternative definitions or explanations and when the dominant view becomes the everyday language of communication.

3. Defining Mental Health

Work in the field of mental health raised even more questions about the power of definition. Turbulent emotions and feelings are part of the human condition and the expression of these feelings is strongly linked to cultural norms and expectations.

Painful emotion is alarming and can appear as a threat to our sense of stability or general wellbeing. This is also true of physical pain but if an injury occurs to a part of our body, reassurance is available through the ability of a doctor to explain what has caused this. We can understand that we have a fracture, for example, that the treatment will re-set the bone and that the drugs will reduce the temporary pain we will experience. We might also appreciate the capacity of our own body to heal and renew itself.

With distress and emotional pain, the causes are more complex and medical knowledge more limited. The concentration on symptom relief is an aspect of the bio-medical approach to mental illness which tends to define feelings such as anxiety, depression or strong emotions as dysfunctional and almost inconsistent with 'normality'. Medical diagnosis of physical illness could not operate without the conceptual framework of defined 'abnormal' and 'normal' states, although even in this field, the boundary between the two are often contested as research in particular specialities reveals new understanding.

In the evaluation of the Tranquilliser Support Group one member described what was special about the group for her:

'It did more for me than all the psychiatrists and all the tranquillisers in the world because it was plain ordinary people that spoke your language... they aren't going to set aside an appointment, its a casual kind of help and nobody is in authority, you are all one to one. I feel that doctors and nurses make me feel inferior, they are in authority and I am nothing. Along there you can let yourself go and cry if you want to cry and panic if you feel like panicking and swear – do all the things that you can't do anywhere else, even in front of your husband and kids, you can go along and shout at everyone if you want to.'

(Project Report 1986)

There is only a small proportion of mental conditions which are directly caused by brain damage, deterioration or disease. Powerful emotions, particularly fear, cause physical effects such as panic attacks, breathlessness, lack of concentration, sweats, irritability, palpitations, inability to sleep and so on, and much medical treatment is directed at these physical manifestations of distress or fear. In fact it is the symptoms themselves which define the 'illness'. For example, a combination of them is diagnosed or defined as depression. Anti-depressants or tranquillisers are prescribed as the treatment to subdue these symptoms and then the patient is expected to feel well again.

For example, the stresses of coping with a new baby are demanding in themselves in a society which gives little support to new mothers but in discussions with local women, it seemed as though these stresses were sometimes compounded by the treatment offered. Once a woman is diagnosed or defined as suffering from post-natal depression and admission to hospital occurs, this triggers off a succession of extra pressures. She firstly has to deal with seeing herself as a mental patient, with all the associated fears, distress and anxiety that this label engenders. She might well be separated temporarily from her baby in hospital and then have to deal with the effects of this. She and the child might have trouble relating to each other or she may feel guilty for failing as a mother. Family and friends might also be anxious and withdraw, emphasising the women's isolation, at a time when she needs most caring for in a human, loving fashion. The drugs she is given often make her feel strange and out of touch with reality and not able to respond well to her child. Her emotions and thoughts might not find expression and in this sense the treatment begins to become part of the problem.

'looking back on the effects the drugs gave me, they gave me normality for a couple of weeks and then after that I felt worse than I did before I had started taking them. That's when the doctor would put up the dosage and then the cycle would begin again, after another couple of weeks. My husband felt I was a hypochondriac because there was always something wrong with me but in fact it was the side-effects of taking anti-depressants and tranquillisers. I felt very confused and dopey. I always felt sick, my mouth was always dry, I sweated a lot and my whole body trembled. I walked around like a zombie for months. My marriage also suffered because I was feeling sedated all the time and I couldn't be bothered to talk to him as I was so withdrawn.

When my baby woke up during the night for a feed I was seldom able to get up for him because I could never waken up. I had nightmares all the time and my husband was left to do everything. Tablets can help as long as there is something else to offer, such as a support group such as ours or individual counselling. Women must be allowed to talk about their feelings rather than being doped up all the time. It was very hard to come off the tablets in the end as I had been on them for so long. They were my whole life. Everytime I felt bad I would climb into a bottle of valium. It took me 4 years to come off them.'

(Project Report 1991)

Implicit in the diagnosis or definition of mental illness is the message that the emotions and feelings that people are experiencing and expressing are 'abnormal' or 'wrong' and that the treatment – usually with drugs, will cure the illness and stop the symptoms occurring. These states can be deeply distressing and can be relieved by drug treatment. However, for many people the definition and assumptions behind it echoed their own worry about the abnormality of such feelings and after medication there would be repeated anxiety about whether they would return – as though they were suffering from a 'cancer of the mind' that could break out again. The definition without explanation did not offer any support or reassurance that although extremely frightening and confusing, sometimes feelings of fear, anxiety or depression might be entirely expected given a particular situation or life experience or that very often they are a normal human reaction when people are under threat or feeling out of control.

Psychotropic drugs were also seen as reducing the capacity for expression and many people felt that their usefulness was limited.

'They held inside the way I felt about the birth of my first bairn, the way I felt about her, you know, it just kept it deep down.'

(Project Report 1986)

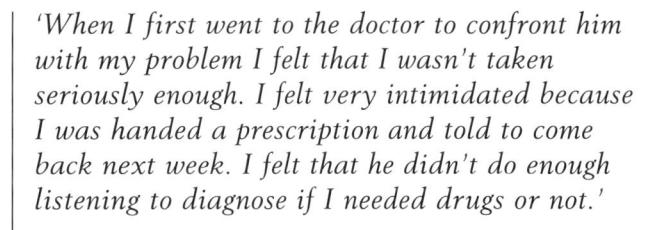

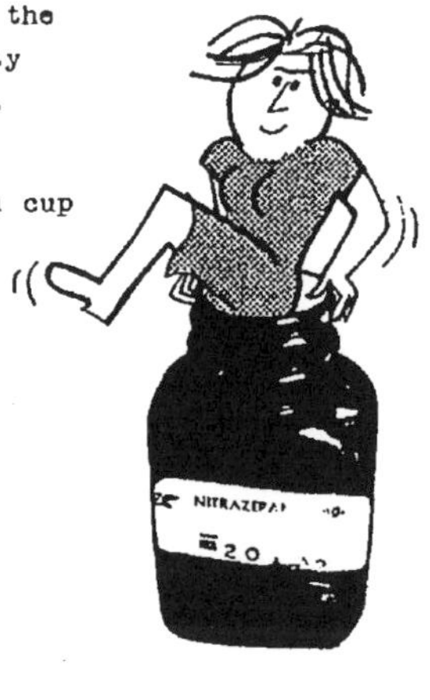

'When I first went to the doctor to confront him with my problem I felt that I wasn't taken seriously enough. I felt very intimidated because I was handed a prescription and told to come back next week. I felt that he didn't do enough listening to diagnose if I needed drugs or not.'

(Project Report 1991)

Working alongside people in the Stress Centre, the tranquilliser groups and the post-natal depression group, many of whom suffered from panic, anxiety and depression, demonstrated that a calm and reassuring response, coupled with some factual information about panic attacks was often enough to help people feel some immediate relief. Reassurance that people were not 'going mad' but that their bodies were reacting physically to some sense of danger, gave them the knowledge to begin to understand a little more about the complex link between our physical and emotional selves. It was then possible to explore the possible reasons for why they might be feeling afraid. Listening to someone expressing their sadness or grief about an aspect of their life offered human comfort and solidarity and enabled them to begin to work out what help they might be able to get in tackling this in more depth.

However in contact with the psychiatric services, these emotions and feelings often became 'symptoms'. These symptoms were what you had when you suffered from mental health problems or mental illness. Once their symptoms had been defined as a form of

First leaflet of the Tranquillisers Group.

Trouble with Tranquillisers?

A small group of women have been meeting and talking about the problems caused when trying to come off tranquillisers such as valium, attivan, librium etc.

We would like to get together with other people in the area who would be interested in tackling this problem together and supporting each other through difficult times.

So we are holding a PHONE-IN WEEK - OCT.29th-NOV.2nd

MONDAY TO FRIDAY 2pm - 7pm

TELEPHONE US ON 551 2556 AND FIND OUT MORE!

We are holding our first meeting on Monday 12thNov between 1.30 and 3.00pm in the Royston/Wardieburn Community Centre, Pilton Drive North. (In the back meeting room)

Come along for a chat and a cup of tea.

mental illness, and themselves as mentally ill, people felt that they entered a new category in society. People spoke about how alienating it was to have a 'psychiatric' label. Neighbours start to act differently, potential employers make excuses for not employing you. Even within the family or close relationships, a wariness develops and you are treated carefully, in case you get upset. Not telling you things, not letting you take responsibility – in a sense being treated like a child. This re-enforced the feeling of being outside normal adult activity and of having little control over the situation. When communications and relationships are filtered through such an overprotective or anxious attitude it serves to increase a sense of isolation and social exclusion, and emotion becomes suspect. People, even close partners, become anxious anytime an emotion such as crying or agitation is expressed, even when these might be entirely appropriate. In these circumstances self-esteem and confidence are so reduced that it can feel unsafe to voice feelings which might only be seen as symptomatic of your illness, not as a real communication.

Many people spoke about their feeling that the interaction with such professionals was often a conversation about how they were feeling but only in terms of whether to increase or decrease their medication. In other words to see how well the drugs were working. A MIND survey of people who had experienced the psychiatric service also identified this problem for patients in their interaction with professionals.

'Patients' communications or expressions of feelings are thus only seen as revealing symptoms, or the progress of the drug treatment, not in terms of them being personally meaningful'.

(Rogers, Pilgrim, Lacy 1993)

Implications for Practice

This effort of hiding real feelings and feeling alone with a fragile understanding of what was going on, was a great strain for many people and it introduced an extra layer of stress, compounding the feeling of alienation and isolation. The constrained and slightly 'unreal' relationships which developed with family and professional workers after being diagnosed as mentally ill, acted to re-enforce a sense of being 'abnormal'.

'dominant groups have a great deal invested in people staying in the correct categories.... It is therefore important that fixed and repressive aspects of categories are challenged as part of strategies of resistance'.

(Meekosha 1993)

In relation to mental health there may be some convenience in people being seen as 'dysfunctional' or 'mentally ill' rather than seeing the level of emotional distress as a possible consequence of social and economic policies, as a result of inequalities of gender, race, sexuality or class, or as a result of abuse.

Work with people who were experiencing mental health problems concentrated on helping people to meet others who had a similar experience, creating a supportive and safe environment which respected the whole person, encouraging people to develop their own 'voice' – their understanding of why they had become ill and providing opportunities for them to critically examine the way mental health is defined in our society. The particular educational role of the worker here is examined in later chapters. In an evaluation of the Stress Centre, the researcher Lisa Curtice highlighted the importance members of the Centre placed on some of these aspects.

'This support from other people in the group was itself a rewarding experience and provided comfort. A sense of feeling understood seems to have been a common experience. One result was that people felt able to show their emotions and to express negative feelings – "Alright to cry there"; "To show your feelings without being frightened"; "Knowing you can have all sorts of feelings, bad and good, and you are able to say how you feel and you have the right to do so without feeling you are a bad person." There was a clear sense that people did not need to be afraid that they would be punished for the way they felt. Thus the group's healing work was in part possible because the usual social consequences of mental health problems, stigma and isolation, were reversed.'

(Curtice, 1991)

Work with women suffering depression around the time of childbirth also revealed the same prioritising of this quality.

'It's a chance to talk through things and feel normal. You do find the answer yourself with a bit of encouragement to talk.'

'I have discovered, through talking to other women that I am not the only one to feel this way.'

'One of the biggest fears is that you are the only one who suffers from it.'

(Project Report 1991)

Conclusion

The process of working with local residents in identifying local concerns and issues is the first stage in a community development strategy. The examples offered here attempt to show that the way health is understood and defined is a complex process. The act of exploring and encouraging people's own agenda, getting below the surface, and questioning everyday assumptions, defines a particular educational role and challenges the fallacy of the 'non-directive' worker. The community development worker in the health field does have an agenda – the agenda is to provide opportunities for people to express their own views, and to question everyday assumptions, explanations and definitions, particularly where they differ with people's own experiences. In a field where official definitions can exert a powerful influence over the content of communication, workers have to be wary of colluding with the dominant views, especially when these have the capacity to oppress people or exclude them from mainstream society.

In the current climate within the health service quick appraisals of the health 'needs' of different groups in the population through questionnaires or one-off focus groups are a regular feature. These methods may have their uses but the responses will be circumscribed by the way health is defined. The impact of social relations on communication is not a new concept but it needs to be addressed, particularly in the field of mental health when issues of power and knowledge and their impact on meaning are so interwoven.

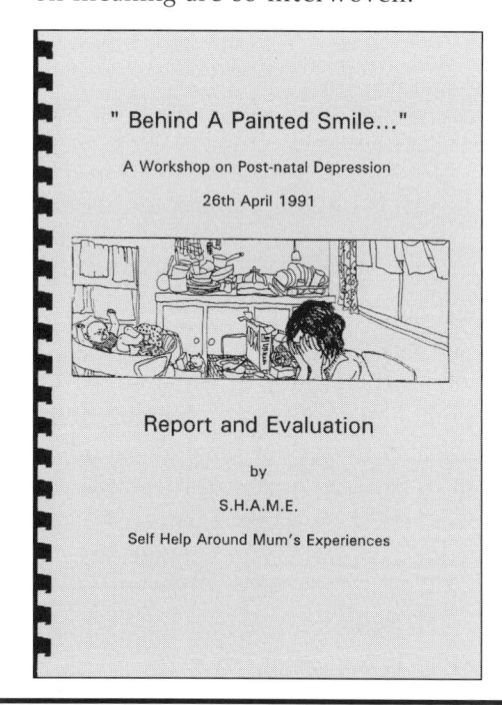

" Behind A Painted Smile..."

A Workshop on Post-natal Depression

26th April 1991

Report and Evaluation

by

S.H.A.M.E.

Self Help Around Mum's Experiences

References

Blaxter, M (1990) — Health and Lifestyles. Tavistock/Routlege, London

Blaxter, M (1983) — Health Services as a defence against the consequences of poverty in industrialised societies, Soc. Sci. Med., 17, pp 1139-48

Cornwell, J (1984) — Hard Earned Lives: Accounts of health and illness from East London

Health and Wellbeing (1992) — K258 Second level course. Dept. of Health and Social Welfare

Kelman, S (1975) — The Social Nature of the definition problem in health, International Journal of Health Services, 5, pp 609-638

Meekosha, H (1993) — The Bodies Politic – Equality, Difference and Community Practice

Butcher, H et al (ed) (1993) — Community and Public Policy. Pluto Press

Minkler, M, ed (1997) — Community Organising and Community Building for Health. Rutgers University Press, New Brunswick, New Jersey and London

Open University (1992) — Health and Well Being K258S. Dept. of Health and Welfare

Rogers, A, Pilgrim, D and Lacey, R (1993) — Experiencing Psychiatry: users views of services, MIND publications. Macmillan

RUHBC (1989) — Changing the Public Health. Wiley & Sons

Stimpson, G V and Webb, B (1975) — Going to see the Doctor: the consultation process in general practice. Routlege & Kegan Paul, London

Pilton Health Project Reports

Jones, J (1986) — Royston Wardieburn Community Health Project: Final Report

Jones, J and Wynn Williams, C (1988) — Developing the Practice

Curtice, L (1991) — An Evaluation of the Middle House Stress Centre

SHAME (April 1991) — Behind a Painted Smile. Report of a workshop on post natal depression.

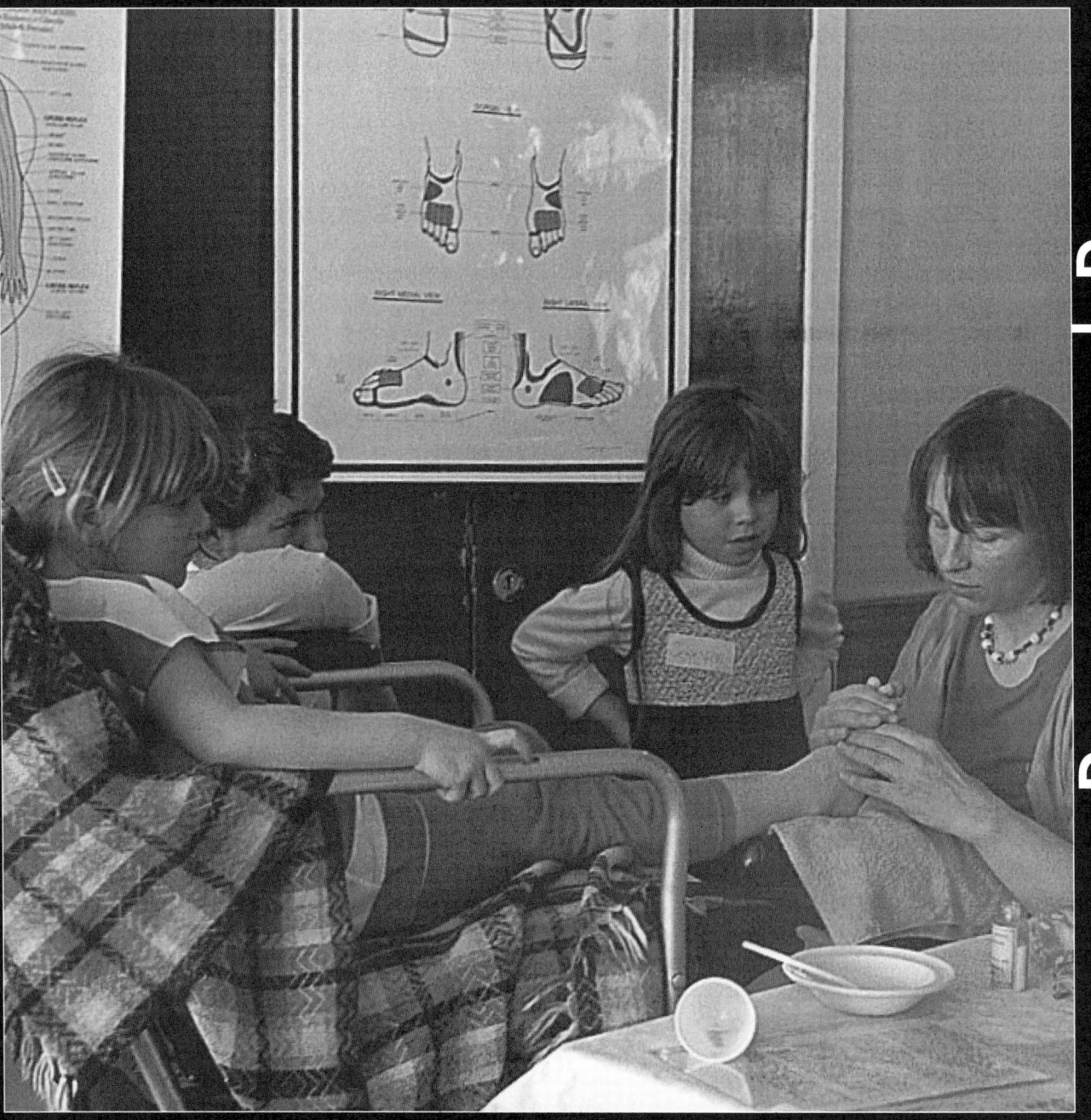

Purpose and Process

Reflexology at a Women's Health Day.

CHAPTER 3

Introduction

Community work involves working and organising alongside local activists and community leaders. The previous chapter illustrated some of the reasons why health issues are not always acted on within communities. The experience of being ill can reduce people's confidence and power and is still viewed as a private matter. Whatever the causes of ill-health, people's first desire is to get well and the emphasis on individual lifestyles has made it hard for the general public to accept health as a political issue. Spontaneous health action groups or activists are not as common as tenants organisations, for example. Community health work is consequently particularly vulnerable to colonisation by professional groups with a variety of different agendas who 'know what the problems are'. Given this context, it is particularly important that we develop an educational practice that encourages local people to identify their own health issues and to take a more critical stance in relation to other agendas. This type of community health practice has to be rooted in people's own interests and life experiences and committed to social and political change. It also needs to be able to offer individual support and practical assistance.

This chapter first of all reflects on aspects of the purpose and process of the work. Drawing on case studies, it then takes two common methods in community work, a single event and work with small groups and examines their potential and limitations. Finally it looks at the interaction between groups and networks as a means of extending participatory democracy.

Clarifying the Purpose

One of the key aims of the Pilton project was to encourage people to identify, explore, investigate, analyse and take action on issues which affected their health through a community development approach. The term community development has always been problematic, it can be seen to be about social change or about social control. The following section outlines the way we interpreted it within the Pilton project during the period 1984-94..

The origins of the Pilton project in the early 1980's meant that our understanding of the term was heavily influenced by the thinking within the community health movement and the women's movement of that period. For example, one of the early community health workers who helped to establish the National Community Health Resource described community development health projects at a SCVO Conference in Crieff in 1987 as follows:

'General characteristics of community development health projects constitute a major commitment by all workers to the tackling of socially created health inequalities and an understanding that a health service cannot provide effective health care in isolation from its most needy users. Community development health projects therefore organise themselves to maximise and validate participation in health issues by people who are amongst the least powerful in our society and who therefore experience poor health and poor health care....

CHAPTER 3

Community development health projects engage head-on with the medical profession, highlighting its centrality and pervasiveness in determining the nature of health and the health service. Users and workers in these projects therefore struggle with issues such as the undemocratic structure of the NHS, the perpetuation of white, male middle-class values as being common currency for all recipients of health care, the increasing alienation from oneself engendered by medical technologies, the individualisation of health and illness and so on.'

(Watt 1987)

Reflecting on this statement from the more fragmented and perhaps politically neutral 1990's, its confident articulation of the social and political nature of community development work in relation to health is a reminder of how far we have travelled over the past decade.

Within the Pilton project, developing our own framework of guiding principles and values (as outlined in the first chapter) helped us to gradually prioritise and shape the work. Having an anchor of principles and values enabled more considered decisions to be taken about which issues to respond to, which groups to work with and which methods would be the most effective. Margaret Whitehead in her work on equity and health observed that if things are inequitable, they are unnecessary and avoidable, unfair and unjust (Whitehead 1990). We found this a helpful and straightforward interpretation of inequity which could directly inform our practice. In the immediate area there was certainly no shortage of examples of inequity and injustice. For example:–

- **research showed a significantly higher rate of attempted suicides in our area and that this was directly related to the high levels of deprivation that people experienced**

- **the proposal to close the childrens' wards and the casualty department in the local hospital when it was known that there was a higher rate of children's accidents and ill-health in the area. The higher accident rate for children in lower income families is known to be linked to higher density housing with less space within the home and inadequate play facilities for children outside. Car ownership and access to private and public telephones were also much lower than other parts of the city, compounding the difficulties parents had in getting access to these services**

- **the siting of the nearby industrial/chemical site in close proximity to a densely occupied working class area. The 'Granton smell' and associated pollution would not have been tolerated in more affluent parts of the city.**

These examples were a constant reminder that the health of local working class people was disproportionately and unfairly affected, in comparison to their middle class counterparts in other parts of the city.

Community development is always a matter of choosing to work with some groups over others. Developing and thinking through a core set of values enabled work to be prioritised with those 'whose living conditions provide them with less material forms of power, such as income, authority over resources or political legitimacy' (Watt and Rodmell 1988) or who were the least powerful and the most marginalised. For example working with older people in residential care, working with big women who felt discriminated against or working with people who had been labelled as mentally ill or had resorted to making an attempt on their life.

Drawing on a social perspective of health meant that issues such as damp housing, the environment, or the poor provision of cheap fresh fruit and vegetables were considered as appropriate areas of work. We saw community development as trying to establish more equitable power relationships between institutions and local groups and this principle of democracy underpinned the aim of encouraging people to become more involved in decisions which affected their lives. It directed us to methods which enabled people to develop a more critical understanding of issues, to develop a strong 'voice' and to support people's right to actively participate in decisions which affected their lives such as the closure of local A&E services. Struggling with ways of giving meaning to these underpinning values through our practice became more important as work developed in all sorts of directions. They gave a sense of coherence in a complex area of work, one in which it is easy to get lost.

Table 1 shows an example of some of the different activities and topics that the project was involved in over some years.

Table 1
Pilton Health Project

Small Groups
Women and Health
Housing and Health
Courses for the Elderly
Family Matters
Food and Families
Middle Years Group
Tranquillisers Group
Women and Food
Loss and Depression
Environment Group

Physical Activities
Keep-Fit for Big Women
Relaxation sessions
Outings/walks
Pensioners Swim Club
Pensioners activities

Surveys
Survey of local shops
Cervical screening
Local Health Survey

Participatory Structures
Pilton Elderly Forum
Clinic Users Group
Listening Ear Mental Health Forum

Campaigns
Feet First Chiropody Campaign
Western General Action Group
Pilton Environment Group

Events
Tranquillisers Open Day
Women's Health Days
Pensioners Conference
Local Conference
'Changes in the NHS' Scottish Conference
'Minor Tranquillisers, Major Problems'

Establishing Local Services
Stress Centre
Counselling service
Pilton Elderly Project
Barri Grubb Good Food Project

Making slide tape programmes and videos
'Who Knows Best?' – feeding and weaning babies
'Home Sweet Home' – damp housing and health
'After You leave the Surgery' – experiences of psychiatric services
'The Granton Smell' – the Pilton Environment Group Campaign

Methodology

As more clarity developed about the purpose of our work it made it easier to decide which methods would be most effective.

Are we wanting to involve new people or to support a group towards independence? What are we trying to achieve with a small number of people working together over weeks or months, compared to a larger single event? How do we create a culture of respect for individuals' own knowledge and opinions? How do we shift the balance of control and power to local residents? What is the role of the worker in each case? Is it to be the educator, the trainer or the facilitator? Is it to be supportive or challenging? When do we bring in outside expertise and how do we do this?

Clarifying these sorts of questions helped us think about the best way of working with people.

Two case studies follow which try to show the progression of local issues through two of the most common community work methods – running single 'events' and working with small groups.

Case Study 1. Women's Health Days

The idea of joining the intimacy of a small group does not appeal to all. It will suit some people but exclude others. Day events allow people to dip their toes in the water and try out things, without too much commitment. Women's Health Days have been a popular feature of community health work and the Pilton project, in collaboration with the local community education team, held three such days over the years. They serve a number of objectives in relation to community health work:

- Making new connections
- Demonstrating a different approach to health issues
- Identifying issues and future work
- Encouraging solidarity between groups

Making new connections

Firstly, they are a good way of making connections with a large number of people in the community, No matter how many well printed leaflets or posters are produced about a group or project, there will still be the comment – but I didn't know about you! Many people like some personal contact before they cross the door or become involved in a new organisation. There are also, always networks that remain unknown, even after years of working in a neighbourhood, and these large events offer an opportunity to break out of the familiar channels of communications and make different connections.

They can provide a platform for local groups to get more publicity for themselves or the issue or campaign, and draw more people into the activities they are running. Lastly, like any social event in a community they provide an informal setting for individuals to make new connections with each other and enjoy the sense of a community gathering. Supporting the informal interaction by providing food, some entertainment, places to sit and chat with tea and coffee is almost as important as the formal programme.

Demonstrating a different approach to health

People's first impressions of a project or group might be through such an event and so the way it is organised, for example, having a good crèche, the issues that are being addressed and the atmosphere, are all important in encouraging people to become involved. More than words these details can demonstrate in action the accessibility of a project, what and who it cares about, what it is willing to support, how it works with local people and how it tackles things.

They can demonstrate an active model of participation. Health 'Days' can sometimes be full of well meaning professionals offering advice and leaflets which carry their educational message into the community. These can be very useful in making a range of information available but the methods employed in organising such an event from a community development perspective would serve a different purpose. If local people are in charge of key planning roles, running workshops or giving presentations, it conveys a message of inclusiveness, of valuing people's own knowledge and increases the likelihood of other people becoming involved as active participants rather than passive consumers, not only on the day but in the future.

Presenting some of the social, environmental or economic determinants of health through a workshop or exhibition, demonstrates concretely an approach to health issues which draws from a social model of health. Serious issues can also be presented in an entertaining and accessible way. For example, for one of the Womens' Health Days, a local arts group, the Muirhouse Festival Association ran an interactive drama sketch which involved two women in an obstacle race, battling with obstacles which stood in the way of them accessing good ante-natal care, to the cheers and laughter of the audience.

Identifying Issues and Future Work

These events stimulate discussion and debate, both formally through workshops or more

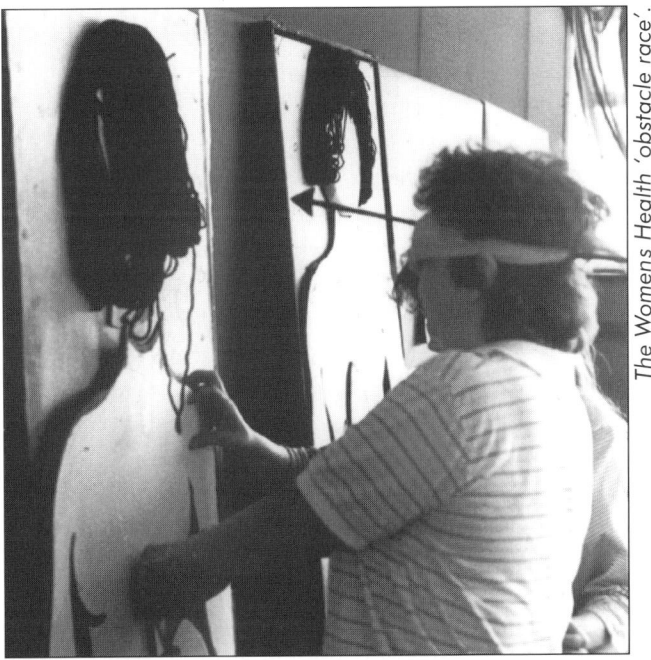

The Womens Health 'obstacle race'.

informally over a cup of tea, about key concerns or issues. These need to be noted in planning future work. For example, the difficulty women had in using the colposcopy services or going for a cervical smear was expressed by women coming to a Women's Health Day. Workshops included topics such as woman and depression, relaxation, and dance as well as an opportunity for women learn to take their own blood pressure to find out what it is. A very approachable local woman doctor had offered to be there so that women could talk informally with her about cervical screening or even have a cervical smear if that was what they wanted. The project report at the end of that year noted the following:

'The way people find out what they want to know is obviously complex. People tended to be drawn to the more positive aspects. Learning about relaxation can make us feel well whereas certain types of screening or information can tell us we might be ill and can therefore arouse some anxiety. There was a big difference between the active interest women had in finding out about their blood pressure, compared to their apparent disinterest in cervical screening. This led the workers to explore these differences and talk about them to local women. Other factors were seen to be important. For example, the screening techniques involved (in taking blood pressure and cervical screening) are very different, one is visible, one is not. One is invasive, examining a very private, sexual part of a women's body and the other is less threatening. The knowledge that one has got high blood pressure is less frightening than if one has got cancer. These observations give an indication as to why women find cervical screening difficult. Leaflets and information put across by the Health Board stress the details of what is involved in a simplistic and cheerful manner, as though it is simply another test. The fears that lie behind the reluctance to be screened or to attend colposcopy clinics are not addressed. If preventive screening is to be accessible to more women, then these factors would need to be taken seriously.'

This issue was noted and eventually worked with through the Well Woman Investigation Group, some time later. They devised a questionnaire and interviewed over 150 women about their experiences of cervical smear and colposcopy services and produced a report 'We Think It's Worth It!' (1992).

Encouraging solidarity between groups

Contemporary society has seen the rise of single issue groups and the impact of consumerism has encouraged 'boxed' identities in order to find new markets, built around particular categories, such as age. These two phenomena can combine in ways which can create divisions between groups and within the wider community. Single events which attract participation from a wider public can provide a useful public forum to demonstrate a different reality – a chance to break out of these limitations and examine common issues or common experiences. For example, reflecting on the first Women's Health Day, it was apparent that it had attracted a majority of younger women. In planning for the second, the involvement of older women was deliberately sought by making a short video with four local women in their 60's and 70's who had been actively involved in community life. The video, which they showed on the day, was about their own experiences such as giving birth to their children at home and their impressions of the health services before and after the National Health Service was established. This provided a link with past generations and by providing an historical perspective of the impact of changes in the NHS and in health policy on the lives of women. It re-connected women with their common experiences in dealing with the health service and encouraged a more critical awareness of the whims and fashions of policy makers.

However, although we were alert to ageism, at that particular time in the late 1980's we were still ignoring issues of race and disability due to our own ignorance and lack of awareness. It was some years later before we began to address the ways in which other groups were experiencing social exclusion.

This type of one-off event therefore served various purposes in terms of people's involvement with health issues, each of which had its own value. Women came for all kinds of reasons. They might have been interested or already involved in the topics or things being offered on the day. They might have been curious about what they would find or they simply might have had nothing better to do that day and there was a crèche for their child. There are therefore all kinds of unforeseen opportunities which might develop. Alison Gilchrist, writing about the importance of networking, labels this activity 'serendipity and strategic opportunism' – making the most out of spontaneous developments which can arise from such an event (Gilchrist 1995).

Apart from the unforeseen opportunities, this kind of event can promote community development values in relation to health; publicise the areas of work that are being undertaken with local women; strengthen alliances with other community workers, agencies and individual health professionals who want to be more accessible to the community; and provide the opportunity for information sharing, networking and identifying local issues that can be pursued in the future. So rather than being viewed as pleasurable but isolated events, they need to be seen as an integral part of the overall community development process.

Case Study 2. Working with small groups

Working with people in small groups provided the energy which directed the whole project but they were all different in terms of membership and content. They ran for different lengths of time, they were different in size and they used different methods, according to their particular objectives. Discussion groups were the most effective way that issues were initially explored. These were usually run for a specific number of sessions, for example 6-8 meetings, ending with a review and 'where do we go from here' session.

Using the popular education methods described in a later chapter, the role of the worker would

Table 2 gives an example of the type of groups, the topics being pursued and their lifespan.

Table 2

Type of Group	Frequency of Meetings	Topics Discussed/Work undertaken
Discussion		
Family Matters	6 weekly sessions	Bringing up children under pressure
Women and Health	8 weekly sessions	Stress, our shape, talking to doctors
Middle Years	1/week for a year	Menopause, relationships, ageism/ageing
Older residents	6 weekly sessions	Stiffness, exercise, cooking own lunch
Self-help Groups		
Women and Food	2 grps over 2 yrs	Feelings and food
S.H.A.M.E.	weekly over 4 yrs	Depression around childbirth
Loss & Depression	4 sessions only	Sharing feelings around bereavement
Tranquillisers	weekly over 2 yrs	Support, side effects, confidence
Investigation		
Who Knows Best?	weekly for 4 mths	Slide/tape made on feeding babies
Well Woman group	work took 18mths	Designing survey. Interviews/coding
Environment group	weekly for 7mths	Video made/campaigning/pollution
Health survey	weekly for 3 mths	Interviewing/collating data
Campaigns		
Feet First	ran for 8 months	Poor chiropody services
Western General	over 4 years	Closure of casualty/children's wards
Environment	over 18 months	Health effects of local chemical works

often be to pose questions such as – what more would we like to know about this? Where can we obtain the information we want? Do you think this affects other people in our area, or nationally? Do we need to talk to more people locally? Are there groups or organisations already working on this? Do we need to explore more how we feel about this through writing or making a sketch?

As group members identified what needed to happen next, this often led onto another type of group or groups, with a more specific purpose.

The discussion group for older residents, for example, was undertaken in order to make contact and develop links with older people living in sheltered housing who felt cut off from community life. The goal was to reduce isolation and to encourage residents to share information, and to try to influence the services provided in the sheltered housing complex so that residents could have more autonomy.

The Pilton Environment Group was started in order to work with local people in developing a more critical understanding of the health impact of a local industrial complex. The group wanted more specialised information and so a course was organised in collaboration with Friends of the Earth, for them and the wider community. This led to the development of a strong campaigning group whose members made a video about a local chemical works, to inform people more widely about the unhealthy practices that were being allowed to occur and the role of the environmental protection agencies.

The Well Woman Investigation was initiated by the project health visitor as a result of concerns being expressed about cervical screening. It was a way of working with local women, as co-investigators, to check out concerns about colposcopy services that had emerged through other individual contacts, group work and the Woman's Health Day. It enabled members to identify the problem areas, develop skills in designing surveys, interviewing and analysing data as well as compiling information from local women in order to try and change service provision.

All these initiatives provided an experience of collectively tackling local concerns and of transforming individual concerns and troubles into public issues. They usually fell into one of four functional categories – discussion groups, support groups, groups carrying out research or an investigation and groups engaged in campaigns, each playing a part in allowing issues to be progressed from identification, to analysis, and through to some action or change.

The broad process of progressing issues is outlined in Table 3 in order to try and sketch out the way the different types of work interconnect and feed each other while acknowledging that it is often much more complex and messy than this.

The different activities, groups and services that might emerge have value in themselves, some of them remaining as more permanent fixtures. Only a small core of people may follow issues through from beginning to end, but at each stage

Table 3 – Progression of Local Issues

LISTENING FOR 'THEMES' – CONCERNS, ISSUES, STORIES
Health Days, Local contacts, all project activities/contacts, conferences

↓

DEFINING THE 'PROBLEM'/IDENTIFYING THE ISSUE
Surveys, discussion groups, short courses, support groups, workshops, making a video

↓

COMMUNITY ACTION

Practical Support	Local Research	Campaigns	Strengthening Local Voice
Eg. Self-help groups, Barri Grubb, Keep Fit for Big Women, Elderly Project, Training	Eg. Local surveys, co-investigations, research	Eg. Western General Action Group, Pilton Environment Group, Feet First Campaign	Eg. Local conferences Forums, campaigns, Public meetings, Clinic user group

↓

DISSEMINATION/NETWORKING/ALLIANCES
Videos, slide/tape programmes, leaflets, booklets, reports, conferences, seminars, public meetings with other community groups, lectures, talks, study visits to other organisations, teaching, articles, training sessions for professionals, student placements, running workshops, visitors coming to project, working with national organisations

in the process others become involved and the build up of expertise and knowledge is extended and shared. For example, the Western General Action Group who ran their campaign to retain local casualty services for over five years, had a strong core group of 10-15 members but at different points in the campaign, would be supported by a wide range of people involved in all the other activities outlined here, as well as hundreds of people in the wider community.

As some of the individual stories show in the last chapter, there is a constant movement in and out of groups – some people leave and become involved in another development, some leave for a while and then return later. During the natural ebb and flow of these interactions, a community project can act as a useful 'holding place' for issues which might need to be put on one side for a while, until there are more people interested or available to continue the work. The choice of methods will enable issues to be tackled in a variety of ways – to be opened up so that more people become involved, to be explored in more depth, to encourage alliances, or to find an immediate solution.

The different stages shown in the life of the Tranquillisers Group gives a flavour of the different ways in which people participated, the different methods used and the different roles the worker undertook.

\multicolumn{4}{	c	}{**The Come Off It! Tranquilliser Group**}
TIMESCALE	**STAGES**	**METHODS**	**ROLE OF WORKER**
Jun 1984	1. IDENTIFYING ISSUES	Women's Health Discussion Group Programme decided by women	Creating opportunities for issues to be identified, To open up agenda
	2. FORMING GROUP	Working with 2 women from above group, visiting other groups, writing leaflets together	Working alongside, finding information, building expertise, giving value to women's knowledge/experience
Nov 1984		Running phone-in	Working alongside
	3. FIRST GROUP MEETING	2 women take lead at first meeting (12 attended)	Advice on planning Support
	4. DEVELOPING THE 'COME OFF IT' GROUP	Programme planned by members, reflection/action pattern, individual group members giving talks to GP's, CPN's etc	Encourage participation Educational support, confidence/ skill building
Nov 1985	5. STARTING SECOND GROUP	Training for members	Educational/supportive
	6. LINKS WITH WIDER NETWORKS/ NATIONAL ORGANISATIONS	Holding Open Day to link with Scottish groups, writing booklet – 'Tranquillity Without Tranquillisers' Organising Scottish conference with SAMH	Broaden issue, make contacts, help in planning, helping reflection/action cycle, Educational Raising wider awareness of issue
Nov 1986	7. DEVELOPING USER-LED LOCAL SERVICE	Review Away Day	Help group to 'look upstream' Plan a preventive service, exploring potential funding resources
	8. STARTING LOCAL MIDDLE HOUSE STRESS CENTRE	Employing 2 local women to work alongside project worker, holding members meetings	Support, to share and develop different perspectives, training for management role

In 1991 a purpose built, member controlled Pilton Reach Out Project (PROP) with 4 staff opened its doors to the community

CHAPTER 3

This example also gives an indication of the different outcomes of the work over time. For the individual it would be a gain in confidence and a reduction in tranquilliser use. It would also be about personal development – running groups, developing skills or gaining employment. It might also offer experience in managing local services.

For the community the work created support groups and the development of the Middle House Stress Centre, an informal resource which eventually expanded into a purpose built centre, Pilton Reach Out Project with more permanent staffing.

Lastly the work helped to widen debate and provide an alternative view of the prescribing and use of tranquillisers.

Self-help groups – limitations and potential

A criticism of groups which run for a long time is that a dis-empowering dependency is created. This can easily happen if there is no longer term strategy which supports people in taking control themselves.

Why do some groups change and develop, take on new members, begin to tackle issues effectively, run their own affairs and gain in confidence? Why do others remain more 'static', surviving with the same core number of participants over many months or years, apparently resistant to any changes suggested and seeming to continue to need worker support?

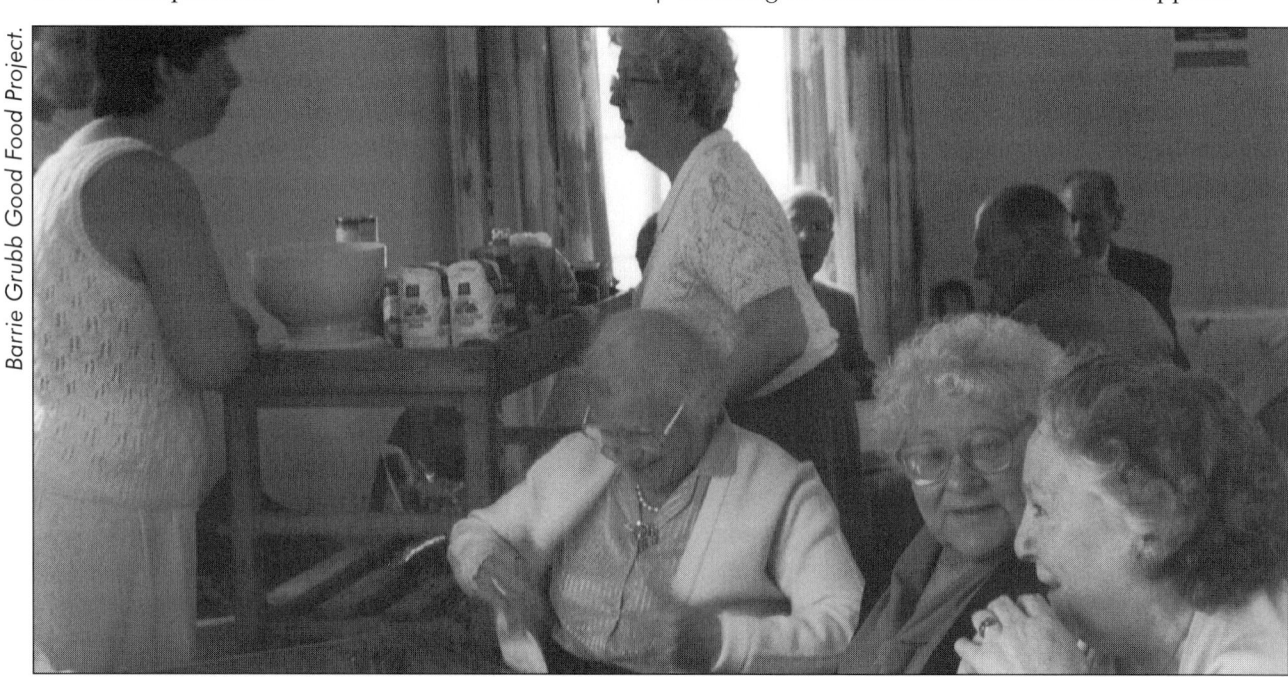

Barrie Grubb Good Food Project.

What is the value in each and what does this tell us about the role of the worker?

One of the characteristics of community health work is that many of the issues that bring people together are often personally and emotionally stressful. Ill-health or lack of access to good health care affect people very deeply. Many people become involved in health groups in order to feel better physically and emotionally and to reduce the feeling of social exclusion or isolation. The implication of this for practice is that the facilitation of the supportive and self-help element within groups is one of the key aspects of the work. However, given that many other professional workers – community psychiatric nurses, health visitors, psychologists, and social workers as well as voluntary groups would also see themselves as running support groups and self-help groups, what is the distinctive contribution of a community development approach?

In an analysis of the different strands within the community health movement, Watt outlined the different roles played by self-help groups and how they are perceived by health professionals. She suggests that self-help groups can be seen as supplementary, complimentary or challenging in relation to traditional forms of health care, depending on the topic they are involved with and the way they act. For example a breast cancer support group will be regarded by the medical profession positively – supplementing their own work. Health professionals will support such groups, sometimes termed 'defensive', often offering their professional expertise, referring patients and even sometimes help in fund-raising. Groups which want to take more responsibility for their own health, as long as it is in accordance with current thinking, such as fitness groups, will also be seen as complimentary. Groups which wish to challenge traditional forms of treatment, for example a mental health users group which wants to question existing forms of medication will be viewed with more suspicion and seen as oppositional. These can be viewed as part of a history of 'offensive' self-help.

Watt saw community development health projects as focusing more specifically on empowerment. To this end they were more likely to be involved in self-help groups which aimed to reduce people's sense of their own powerlessness and to increase equity and access, activities which often proved a challenge to medical hegemony, rather than supporting the status quo (Watt 1986). Labonte also stresses the difference between support group work which concentrates on healthy or equitable power relations within the group and community development work which focuses on developing equitable power relations between community groups and institutions (Labonte 1997).

The underlying values and the educational role of the community development worker in the health field gives this form of group work its distinctive quality and the combination of these support, educational and action roles, one of its major challenges. Although there is a tendency for workers to be drawn to one particular role, sometimes as a consequence of their own experience, qualification and background, effective work depends on a combination of these elements. This does not mean that a single worker has to carry all these different and sometimes difficult roles, but that these different elements are recognised and supported where possible, sometimes using outside expertise or drawing from the skills of workers in the local area.

'Unless the right of groups to lobby for changes in government policy is recognised and supported in health promotion funding policy, the self-help ethos restricts to a personal level problems that have both personal and political dimensions.'

(Labonté 1997)

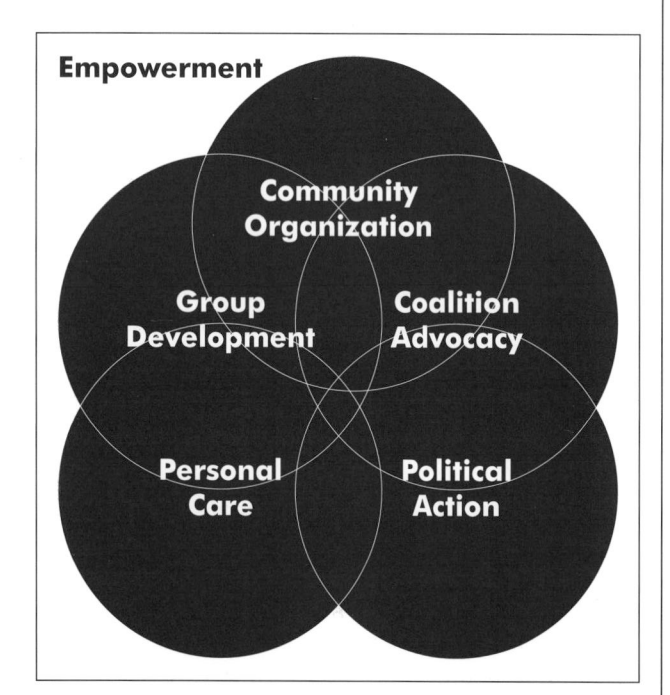

Empowerment

- Community Organization
- Group Development
- Coalition Advocacy
- Personal Care
- Political Action

(Labonté 1998)

From the Pilton project's experience, groups where there was an emphasis on action but a neglect of the supportive function often lost members – with a few stalwarts left doing all the work; in groups where the focus remained on surface problems, without any articulation or critical reflection, people's creative energy became blocked, there was often a slow decline in membership and there was little sense of direction; and in groups where there was a concentration on analysing problems but taking no action, a sense of frustration and boredom. The emphasis on each role will depend on the group, the issues people are concerned about and the stage of development.

The strategy adopted in the Tranquillisers Group included many different roles at different times. Initially there was a focus on exploring issues thoroughly, and checking them out with a wider circle of people to make sure that they genuinely reflected peoples' concerns. This ensures support, commitment and interest. Taking time over this process allowed mutual support to be built up, more analysis and discussion of the issues and ensured that they 'belonged' to local people, not to workers, and emphasised and affirmed people as active 'subjects', not 'objects'.

Building confidence and trust through small 'successes' – or achievable gains at each stage, creates a strong base that enables people to branch out, to take control of the development, take issues further and take more risks. Starting with small but solid building blocks enables larger structures and organisations to flourish. From this perspective, it does not matter in the early stages, if only two or three people are concerned about an issue. For the reasons outlined in the previous chapter, health issues are often unarticulated and the few people who do speak out, the tip of the iceberg. Sometimes this can dishearten workers who have expectations of larger turnouts at their first community meeting. This sense of failure can be picked up by the few people attending so they in turn feel disappointed and might not return. This is a missed opportunity as often these small group meetings allow more to be said and listened to with attention.

In our experience, the people who become involved at this initial stage often became active co-workers. For example, when organising a first local meeting they would play a crucial role in helping people relax as they saw it was not going to be dominated by professional workers, by sharing their own first hand experience as a way of setting the agenda and embedding this right from the beginning. This also enabled relationships and trust to develop.

In an economic climate which wants a quick return of investment in the form of 'results', this style of community development work will suffer. As workers, we need to make this underlying practice more visible, by describing the process more clearly and developing and articulating a clear rationale for its role in community development practice, despite the push to concentrate on speedy outcomes and numbers. We need to re-frame the parameters of evaluation to include some of the stages and processes as 'outcomes' and in the process re-educate funders about what to expect from the community development process. For example, members beginning to take over the running of a group can be a legitimate first stage goal and can be measured through qualitative evaluation methods.

Training and support for local unpaid workers is essential, not only for their own development but in helping the group move forward. As a matter of principle, the Pilton project always tried to secure sessional payment for people taking on any regular commitment and eventually to create more secure employment. Apart from the counselling service where local people preferred that the workers came from outside the area, all of the separate services and initiatives that developed had a majority of local people employed in them.

The impact of change on people's lives who moved from being a member of a support group, to facilitating a group or to becoming a paid worker was considerable and not always positive. Changing roles and relationships brings other stresses and losses. A series of meetings the project held with local women who had experienced these changes revealed the pressures they had to contend with – from families, partners, neighbours who resented or were alarmed and threatened by their personal development. We were aware how little we had appreciated the difficulties of these changes. The work of Peter Marris drew our attention to the importance of losses, large and small which accompany the process of social change – whether at individual level as described here or at a community level following the effects of slum clearance or the decline of a major industry (Marris 1986). Much community development literature is concerned with the broader social and political process of change. An awareness of the impact of change on people's immediate relationships and sense of identity could help us be more sensitive as workers and create ways to enable people to discuss and acknowledge this process.

The 'Chain Reaction' Process and Participatory Democracy

Written reports on the practice of community development and health show a concentration on descriptive accounts of specific pieces of work but, less on the form of practice which, over time, consciously creates a dynamic and an interaction **between** different types of activities and networks, an interaction which actively supports participatory democracy.

Although the Pilton project's funding was on an annual basis, it was continued without too much insecurity over this ten year period. This enabled it to support and stimulate this broader community development process which can be a vehicle for both extending the opportunities for people to participate and act collectively and for informal, popular education. It can provide a public space for the critical examination, exploration, and articulation of local health issues. As groups grow and develop and different activities occur, there is scope to support and stimulate the interaction and dynamic between them in order to create active networks of interest and solidarity around common issues.

For example, the issue of tranquilliser use was raised by two women in the first group run by the project, a Women's Health Discussion Group. As outlined previously this in turn led to the development of support groups, the publication of an alternative approach to tranquilliser withdrawal, the joint organising of a national conference, culminating in a purpose built, user-run Stress Centre three years later. These initiatives also contributed to the setting up of a local mental health forum.

The same Women's Health Discussion Group also identified damp housing as one of the most important health issues facing them and their families. This led to a second 'spin-off' – the creation of a Health and Housing Group who made the slide/tape programme 'Home Sweet Home' which in turn stimulated Edinburgh University researchers to conduct a local study into the effects of damp housing on health, followed by two further major studies (Martin 1987). The women who were involved in both began to make the connections between inadequate and unhealthy housing, mental health and the prescribing of tranquillisers.

As groups identify issues and change direction or focus, new people are brought in at each stage, extending the learning and the level of participation. This 'chain reaction' process can be seen in more detail in the next case study, charting the activities and events which came out of work with older people. These different activities enlarged the public's perception of health issues facing the elderly and encouraged more people to participate in an active way and make the connection between their personal experiences and wider policy and resource issues.

Case Study 3: Working with Older People

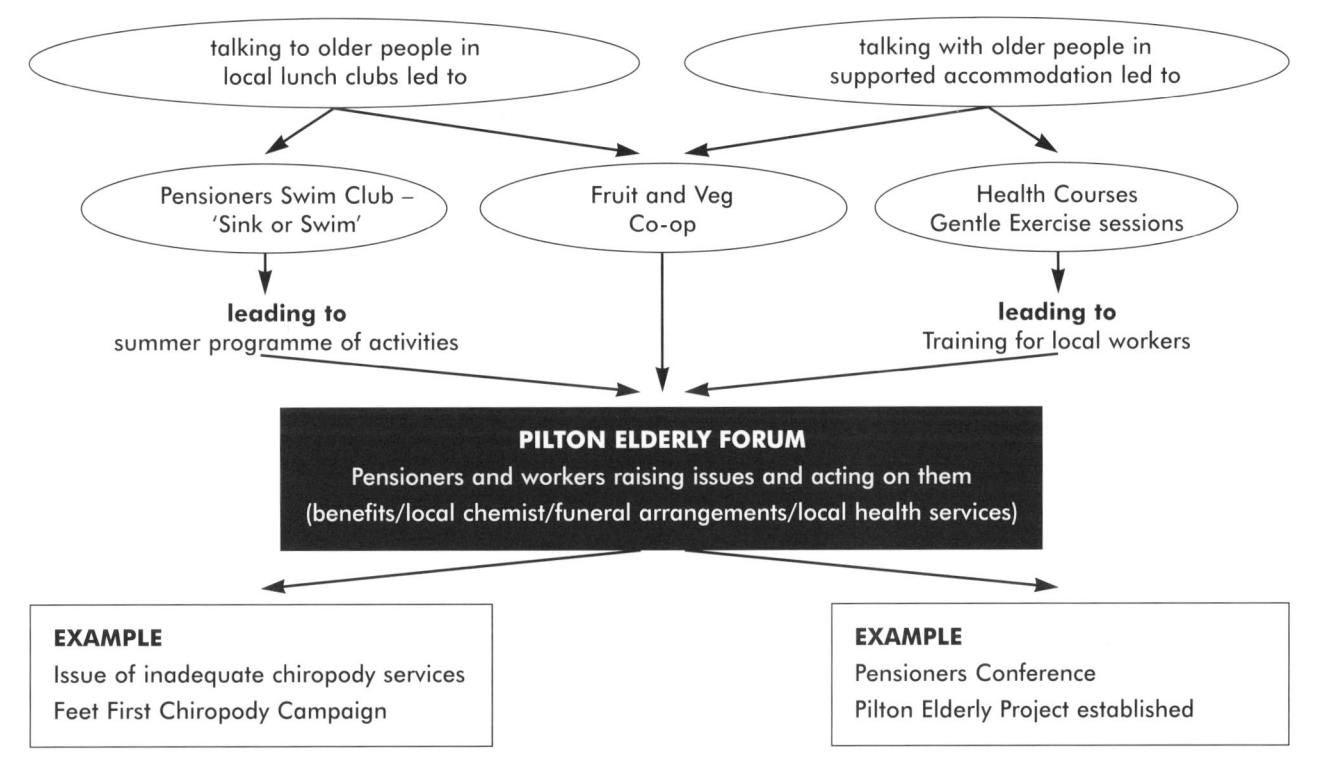

```
talking to older people in          talking with older people in
local lunch clubs led to            supported accommodation led to
        ↓           ↓                      ↓            ↓
 Pensioners Swim Club –       Fruit and Veg         Health Courses
   'Sink or Swim'                Co-op         Gentle Exercise sessions
        ↓                            ↓                     ↓
    leading to                                        leading to
summer programme of activities                  Training for local workers
                                ↓
        ┌───────────────────────────────────────────┐
        │           PILTON ELDERLY FORUM            │
        │ Pensioners and workers raising issues and │
        │              acting on them               │
        │ (benefits/local chemist/funeral           │
        │  arrangements/local health services)      │
        └───────────────────────────────────────────┘
              ↓                               ↓
```

EXAMPLE
Issue of inadequate chiropody services
Feet First Chiropody Campaign

EXAMPLE
Pensioners Conference
Pilton Elderly Project established

The initial work with older people was developing small initiatives in response to issues they had identified – the need for more information and social activity for the residents in supported accommodation; the need to 'do more than play bingo' expressed by women in a local lunch club leading to the 'Sink or Swim' Club; and the need for easier access to small fresh quantities of food leading to the first food co-op. These activities then led onto more and the relationships that developed allowed the workers to be more in touch with a number of common issues facing older people. Discussions ensued as to the best way of tackling these. The idea of a local Forum grew. In collaboration with other local groups and organisations, such as the Pilton Central Association and local community education workers, the health project set up the Pilton Elderly Forum (PEF) pooling our joint experience and networks. This was a way of drawing people together in order to see the common issues that faced them and to provide a means to take action about them. As well as older people living in the area, the local branch of SOAPA (Scottish Old Age Pensioners Association), local professionals such as GP's, district nurses, home helps, health visitors and social workers were also invited to take part.

The Project's role was to encourage a wide representation of different groups across the area to be involved in setting up the Forum through community meetings – to generate an inclusive rather than an exclusive ethos; to ensure that older people set the agenda by taking up key positions such as Chair and Secretary; and encouraging a majority of older people to attend to ensure that the Forum did not become professionally dominated.

After the Forum was established, the project helped to service and maintain it by getting minutes of meetings typed, offering accommodation and refreshments, organising transport and helping to get publicity leaflets produced.

The Chiropody Campaign

The network of groups and relationships enabled issues to be articulated more publicly. For example, the lack of chiropody services was first talked about in the changing rooms of the swimming group and during the health course in the sheltered housing complex. It was brought to the attention of the Forum and a highly successful Chiropody Campaign – 'Feet First' was launched which is described more thoroughly in the following chapter. The campaign in conjunction with the local health council, transformed the inadequate and patchy service into a regular weekly one and in turn attracted other groups in Lothian to take the campaign into their areas.

A Community Conference

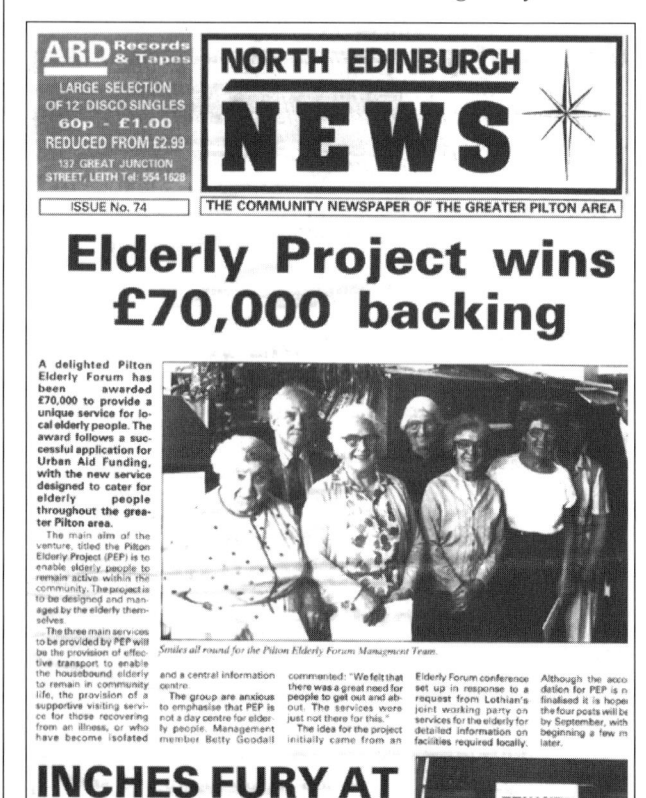

The Forum was consulted over the council's proposed strategy for older people and this prompted the workers to suggest a conference where the proposals could be discussed more thoroughly. As well as producing a response for the council, the thinking and ideas generated from this conference formed the basis of an urban aid application for a local initiative that the Forum put together later that year. This led to the funding of the Pilton Elderly Project – a successful local resource managed by older people which offers transport, information and a befriending service for housebound people

The flat, rather than hierarchical, structure of the Forum with different working groups, prevented a small clique from developing and filtering information from outside – any enquiry of the Forum was brought to the open meeting. This open structure encouraged wider participation from those attending and allowed both for the diversity of local groups so that their individual group interests and identity were protected as well as the means for them to come together around common concerns. At the Forum, representatives from the Scottish Old Age Pensioners (SOAPA) branch, the pensioners swim group or the local district nurses, for example, could maintain their different interests and perspectives but were also able to work across identity and organisational boundaries to develop alliances around particular issues such as the inadequate chiropody services.

Each new development created its own small 'chain reaction', increasing the number of people involved each time and enlarging the network of people who had an interest in the issues affecting the health of older people. The Pilton Elderly Forum provided a structure where these issues could be debated and action taken on them. The Forum also worked with other local organisations and groups on wider issues which affected the whole community, such as the closure of the local casualty department, or the changes in the NHS.

Conclusion

These particular aspects of the community development process have been disentangled in order to examine them more closely. However as stated in the beginning of this chapter, the way they inter-connect and weave together has to be seen as a whole, in context and over a considerable period of time.

Reflecting on this living, dynamic process, two things stand out from the experiences of the Pilton project. Firstly, as discussed in the previous chapter, the way issues are defined, articulated and tackled will have an influence on the levels and quality of participation. Using methods which encourage people to participate in defining, articulating, analysing, reflecting and tackling local health issues are crucial.

The action, reflection cycle, proved a useful tool in much of the work. This constant cycle of 'reflection with ongoing commitment to action' (Kirkwood 1989) is described in more detail in later chapters.

Reflection: Action diagram based on Hope, Timmel and Hodzi, 1984

If issues are defined by outside agencies or organisations which find no resonance with local peoples' experience, then a low level of participation can be expected. This is sometimes called 'apathy'.

Secondly, the whole process of involvement and participation is held together by human relationships. People might well be concerned over particular issues but the process of engaging with these, has to be a satisfying, stimulating or enriching experience. Groups need to feel inclusive, not exclusive and a place where individual views are given serious consideration. The level of participation depends crucially on nurturing positive relationships as well as sometimes supporting individuals and can be directly related to the seriousness and respect given to people's views and opinions and the commitment to jointly exploring the underlying problem. Learning can be a positive experience even if it involves effort and struggle.

One of the characteristics of the Pilton project was a sense of growth and movement despite the fact that issues were progressed over quite long periods of time – sometimes years. As these case studies show, there were relatively few examples of short term work that were not linked in some way to other initiatives as part of a longer term strategy. This was not part of any 'grand plan' at the beginning but more a consequence of a style of work that gradually developed. As workers, we only began to note its significance after working in the area for a number of years. The key elements of this seemed to be the combination of both stability and change.

Stability and consistency were sustained through the strong ongoing relationships that developed between local people and the project and the continuous, collective, building of alternative analyses, the development of a local 'voice' on health matters. The cycles of planning, action and reflection and the range of different initiatives, collaborative work and student placements, energised and stimulated this stable core and brought a regular flow of new ideas and new people into this process.

The example of the development of the tranquilliser group given here, shows how participation can lead to action which can begin to have a real influence on individuals and on the broader debates which need to take place in order to eventually affect policy and practice as well as the creation of more effective services. However the progression and articulation of issues through different strategies and methods is a key role for the community development worker. The value of working at neighbourhood level with small numbers of people need not be written off as 'localism' as long as there is a clear sense of purpose, an ongoing attempt to broaden out the issues, disseminate information more widely, and form outside networks and alliances.

The timescale of this process is crucial and the contention in this chapter is that if resources are made available to support a longer investment in the community development process, then real gains for the health of the community can be made.

References

Watt, A (1987) — The Community Response to Medical Dominance: Room for Movement? Talk given at the SCVO Conference on Community Development and Health in Crieff Hydro

Watt, A (1986) — 'Community Health Initiatives: Clarifying the complexities within the Community Health Movement' paper given at the Conference 'Community Development in Health: Addressing the Confusions'

Whitehead, M (1990) — The Concepts and Principles of Equity and Health. World Health Organisation

Gilchrist, A (1995) — Community Development and Networking, Briefing Paper, No.5. Standing Conference for Community Development and Community Development Foundation publications

Labonte, R (1997) — Community, Community Development and the Forming of Authentic Partnerships in Community Organisation and Community Building, ed, Minkler, M. Rutgers University Press

Labonte, R (1998) — A Community Development Approach to Health Promotion: A background paper on practice tension, strategic models and accountability requirements for health authority work on the broad determinants of health, HEBS and RUHBC. University of Edinburgh

Martin, C J, Platt, S and Hunt, S M (1987) — Housing Conditions and ill-health, British Medical Journal, pp 294 1123

Kirkwood, C & G (1989) — Living Adult Education

Marris, P (1986) — Loss and Change, Revised edition. Routledge & Kegan Paul

Pilton Health Project Reports

Pilton Well Woman Investigation Group (1992) — We Think It's Worth It! – A survey on women's experience of cervical smear and colposcopy services

Conflict and Co-operation

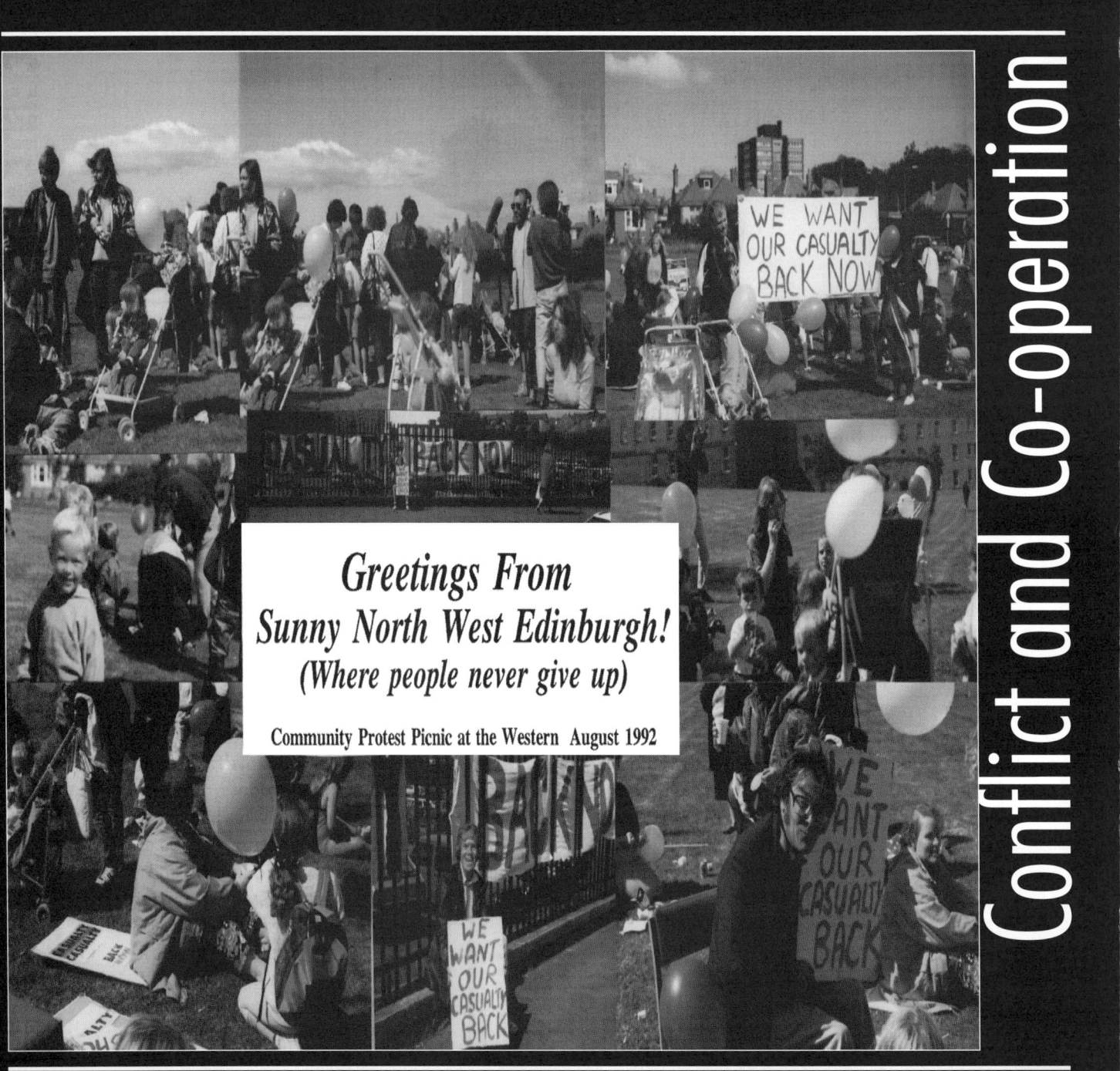

Greetings From Sunny North West Edinburgh!
(Where people never give up)

Community Protest Picnic at the Western   August 1992

Campaign 'postcard' sent to the Health Board.

Introduction

This chapter documents and reflects on the shifts in thinking which took place as we attempted to support local people taking various courses of action. These shifts roughly approximate to the different stages in the early years of the project's life but like all human activity, they interconnect and overlap in many ways. Trying to achieve even small changes in attitudes, in extending representative democracy or in the way health services were planned and provided often felt like trying to plant trees in a desert. It was hard work even to create a small space in the sandy soil, and as fast as people dug, the sand had a habit of slipping down and constantly filling the hole.

Two phases are described, which are sufficiently distinct to use them for the basis of this type of reflection and analysis. During the first phase, when the project was based in a local general practice, we were exploring how far a community development approach could be developed within the context of primary health care. The second phase covers the experience of working from a new base in a local primary school when, with an expansion in funding, the project tried to develop more effective strategies to support local action, largely by developing structures and networks.

The First Phase: Local Action and Primary Health Care

The case studies in this section need to be seen in context. As has been described in the introduction, the health project started its life based in a general practice. One of its aims was to try to encourage GP's to support this type of work and in recognition of their busy workload one of the GP's in the practice was paid an extra sessional allowance to enable them to work with the project. Two issues are used to explore the constraints on moves to change attitudes or service provision. Firstly the prescribing of tranquillisers and secondly, the effects of damp housing on health.

The Prescribing of Tranquillisers

There were three main initiatives in relation to the prescribing of tranquillisers: a self-help group, a conference and a seminar.

The 'Come Off It' Group

This self-help group described in the previous chapter, developed from a core of local people who wished to reduce their dependence on minor tranquillisers and draw attention to some of the harmful side effects. It grew fast and was a very successful group which provided information, advice and support for local people and rather naively perhaps it was assumed that the GP's would welcome this. However, certainly in the beginning there was some hostility and very little support for this group from the practice GP's. This was discussed in the first Project Report in 1986 under the heading 'What are the obstacles to co-operation?'

'Perhaps because this group represented an intrusion into the area of clinical judgement it met

with particular difficulties. As it developed, comments from some of the practice GP's indicated that they felt tranquilliser dependency was not a particular problem, that the group challenged their expertise and judgement in prescribing appropriate treatment for their patients and that patients should tackle this problem with their doctor rather than form groups.'

About a year later the group grew more successful and two of the women doctors began to send referrals. It was, however, supported by the local social work staff, one of whom worked closely with the project worker in its formation. Community psychiatric nurses (CPN's) were also supportive and a community psychiatrist came and gave input to the group on various topics. In general terms the health visitors in the practice felt it was a positive development and one of them joined the group in attending a conference run by MIND in Newcastle. The group went on to produce and write a booklet, 'Tranquillity without Tranquillisers' and over a thousand copies were sold to a range of individuals and support groups but also to a high proportion of health professionals, health visitors and CPN's.

Scottish Conference on Tranquillisers

To widen the debate and connect with the ground swell of interest that the group was aware of and also part of, a national conference was organised together with the Scottish Association for Mental Health entitled 'Minor Tranquillisers, Major Problems'. The key speakers included a local psychiatrist, a clinical psychopharmacologist from Newcastle whose research confirmed the existence of side effects, and a member of the Pilton 'Come Off It!' group. The conference was attended by over 150 people, including health visitors, CPN's, over 40 organisations and many individuals. GP's were invited but only one or two attended. A lot of interest was generated, a report published of the proceedings and an informal network of interested groups was established.

Seminar for GPs

To capitalise on the fact that the researcher from Newcastle was going to be in Edinburgh for the above conference, a seminar was also organised specifically for GP's. The researcher, Dr Heather Ashton was an eminent consultant in clinical pharmacology, who had done extensive research in the early 1980's on the longer term use of minor tranquillisers, the danger of side effects, withdrawal effects and dependency. We felt that GP's particular interests might be submerged in a larger, public conference and so with the help of a consultant community psychiatrist, invitations went out to most GP practices in the North West of Edinburgh and about 12 attended. After her presentation, the senior partner from one of the larger practices commented icily that despite her 'very elegant presentation', in all his years of practice, he had never found side effects or dependency on tranquillisers to be a problem! Given the hierarchies and dynamics within general practice, this dictated the parameters of the discussion which followed. There was no observable response from the GP's after the seminar in terms of communication or referrals although over time some GP's made a small number of referrals to the group.

At this time, in 1985, the number of prescriptions for benzodiazepines in the UK stood at 25.7 million. The conference and seminar need to be seen as part of an increasing lobby for change. The scale of the problem prompted a nation wide protest which eventually became co-ordinated by MIND and the TV programme 'That's Life' leading to a wave of litigation against the drug companies and some doctors (Lacy 1991). Guidelines cautioning doctors about their use of these drugs then emanated from a number of Royal Colleges of Medicine. Since then there has been a steady decline in the prescription rate as these drugs became discredited for their addictive qualities. Evidence from the research establishment caught up with patients' own experience of these drugs and their withdrawal symptoms but it was the threat of legal action which finally turned the tables. The local action taken had little immediate effect but as part of the network of protest across the UK, supported by the media and finally by law, eventually had an impact nationally on the over prescribing of these drugs.

The second issue that we tried to work with was that of damp housing and its effects on the health of children and adults.

Damp housing

Damp housing was an issue which was brought up time and time again in the early days of the project, through many informal conversations on doorsteps and in community centres. It was raised through the first discussion group the project ran and this was tackled in a variety of ways in an attempt to raise awareness that dampness was not a 'private trouble' but a public issue. Links were also made with the city wide tenants movement but this section focuses on the relationship with health professionals. Four initiatives were undertaken.

Making a slide-tape

Out of the women's health discussion group the issue of damp housing was identified as a major concern. Funds were obtained from community education and a tutor taught the women how to take photographs and edit tape recordings. Over a three month period they made a slide-tape presentation to show the effect damp housing was having on their own health and their children's health 'Home Sweet Home'. It covered various aspects of the problem, such as the difficulty getting their children immunised because they always had colds and coughs, their own stress and the cost of having to replace mouldy clothes and keep extra heat in the rooms they were living in. They interviewed the practice GP working with the project, who had a background in public health medicine and was particularly aware of the social influences on health. They interviewed housing officials, trade union representatives and environmental health staff. After meeting with the practice GP and discussing the issue, two further pieces of action were planned. It was felt that more evidence should be gathered to support the tenants claims by monitoring the extent of dampness amongst those patients who reported respiratory problems and that we would interview the medical officers of the Health Board to investigate the medical support for re-housing.

Monitoring health effects

The GP tried to persuade his colleagues to monitor the extent of damp housing amongst patients coming to the practice with respiratory complaints. This involved a simple form that we had drawn up, asking patients for this information over a two month period. The practice meeting rejected this as being too 'political'. It was seen as 'district council business' which might be used by one political party. It was not seen as an issue they should get involved in.

Medical 'lines'

The GP and myself next sought an interview with the medical advisor of the Health Board to discuss the way the health effects of poor housing were interpreted in the assessment and endorsement of medical support for re-housing. The medical advisor merely re-iterated the department's position. Mental stress caused by inadequate or damp housing was not considered to be a 'medical' matter. They merely took account of patients' physical conditions or mobility. Later on in our discussion it was admitted that despite this official position, two thirds of letters sent in by GP's supporting rehousing on medical grounds, referred to the mental stress caused by housing conditions. So GPs themselves were interpreting the mental stress caused by dampness as a medical matter but the official line dismissed this. Even though there are major discrepancies and variations within housing authorities in the use of medical priority to guide allocation policies and procedures (Smith 1990), these different interpretations of what constituted a 'medical matter' illustrate the ambivalence of the profession when it approaches the boundary between bio-medical and socio-political accounts of health.

Forming Alliances

The self-help group arranged to show the local health visitors the tape/slide 'Home Sweet Home' and present their concerns to them,

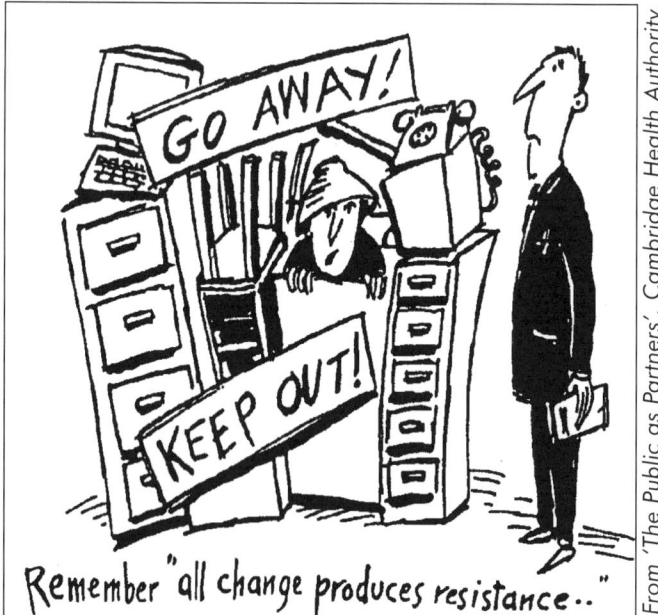

Remember "all change produces resistance.."

From 'The Public as Partners'. Cambridge Health Authority.

particularly with regard to their children's health. The health visitors were supportive of the women's position and expressed their own concerns but clearly felt unable to effect any influence on policy or management or to support the women in any but an individual way. Their response characterised the sense of powerlessness, often experienced by health visitors, which can be seen as a reflection of their position within the medical hierarchy.

Connections were made between the project and the Research Unit for Health and Behavioural Change (RUHBC) at Edinburgh University. The group was invited by the unit to conduct a seminar about dampness and ill health. A robust debate followed the slide/tape presentation, with members of the group taking on a Professor of General Practice who seemed to be suggesting that the state of the area was people's own fault. This type of interaction between local tenants and medical academics was probably highly unusual. It had the effect of encouraging a group of researchers to offer to help research into the effects of damp housing and health although the research that was eventually published portrays the tenants as somehow appearing by magic without any acknowledgement of the community development work that had led to the articulation and the presentation of this issue in so vivid a form. This local research in the Royston/Wardieburn area of Pilton later led to a major piece of research undertaken within 3 cities, (Martin, Platt, Hunt 1987) which has become a key piece of evidence in exposing the social and economic influences on health. It also had the effect of temporarily pushing the District Council to speed up their rehabilitation programme for this area of Edinburgh.

Unfortunately because of the length of time it took, and it being seen as a separate activity, by the time the initial research was available, the housing and health group had gone on to other things, the local tenants group had disappeared and there was no ongoing work between the tenants and researchers. The researchers did however form a successful alliance with the Easthall tenants group in Glasgow which continued to actively campaign and lobby about damp housing and health.

Discussion

These examples show the way in which different types of initiative produced different responses from primary health care staff and other professionals. Although they relate to a particular group of individuals in one general practice at a particular time and place, there are lessons to be learnt from this experience in terms of the relationship between community development and primary health care.

Firstly, some initiatives were supported by primary health care staff if there were common or complementary aims and if what was being asked of them was seen as coming within their professional sphere of influence and expertise. For example, being interviewed, about specific medical conditions or services for the slide/tape presentation, meant that their professional expertise was valued and they were often pleased to share this with wider groups in the community. Any action which implicitly or explicitly challenged their professional areas of judgement and jurisdiction, and therefore status and status relationships were strongly blocked. The reactions in relation to the issue of tranquillisers for example, when it was implied that there was an over-prescribing of tranquillisers, illustrates this particular aspect very clearly – the issue was ignored or there was resistance and even hostility.

Secondly, their support of local initiatives was often dependent on their own position in the health hierarchy. The consultant community psychiatrist for example, who supported the idea of the local self-help group on tranquillisers, the conference and the seminar, and who was sympathetic to community development work, had sufficient status and power to decide on her own area of work. If, like the practice GP, they were dependent on their colleagues approval within a practice team or in attempting to exert influence outside their own territory such as with the district medical officer, these were limiting factors on the amount of support they felt able to offer. Health visitors, whose position in the medical hierarchy is often under the scrutiny of doctors, seem to feel particularly powerless to overtly support any community initiative which implicitly or explicitly challenged medical dominance. They were sympathetic about damp housing but felt powerless to help and did not see their professional role as actively or publicly supporting groups in this way.

Lastly, it appeared that many health professionals found it difficult to support the community's interests when it required them to broaden their perspective, to engage in new areas of practice, or to engage at a political level.

In many ways the reluctance of health professionals to use their professional muscle in the realm of preventative health care at a social rather than an individual level simply reflects the health policy paradigm which has dominated the twentieth century. In the nineteenth century, public health reformers appreciated that disease and illness were caused by poverty and conditions of working and living. In the twentieth century, the rise of bio-medical science led to the belief that this new knowledge would eliminate disease and illness. This was why free and universal access to medical health care was seen to be one of the pillars of the National Health Service. The belief was that medical science would gradually eliminate most ill-health and the demand for health care would be reduced. The discovery of new drugs which could cure tuberculosis, for example, in the 1950's led to a concentration on people coming forward for treatment, while the conditions which allowed tuberculosis to flourish were given lesser status.

In 'In the Clear', a video made about a TB campaign in Pilton in the 1950's, public health doctors are explicit about the way that the medical profession in the UK ignored the evidence about the link between overcrowding **and** TB and turned all their attention to treatment. In Sweden they decided to get rid of their slum housing as well and by the late 1940's they had eliminated slum housing and TB, whereas in Scotland we still had both (Video in Pilton, 1984).

The reaction of the practice GP's to the issue of respiratory disease and damp housing was very similar to the way the medical profession reacted to TB and the link with poor housing conditions, forty years earlier.

When an issue such as damp housing crossed the social/medical boundaries doctors seemed reluctant to act even when it was apparent that the problem was not being dealt with and it was affecting the health of their patients.

The Labour government which came into power in 1997 has indicated a willingness to acknowledge the social, economic and political causes of ill-health but as discussed in future chapters, it will also need to acknowledge the power of the professions in maintaining the status quo, the need for a real shift to preventative and public medicine and the need for a more democratically controlled health service.

Conflicts of Interests

Through these kinds of experiences, there was an awareness of the different conflicts of interests which were blocking change and the limited effectiveness of some of the action that had been taken. It also showed the way the medical profession controls areas of influence. The individual GP's or consultants who wish to be more responsive, or see the need for change or different practice, can be subject to quite considerable peer pressure or even be isolated or marginalised if they persist. The researchers at the RUHBC who explored the health effects of damp housing were subject to pressure to revert to more lifestyle research (Martin 1989), although as academics they might be perceived as having slightly more autonomy. The case of Wendy Savage, the London obstetrician who was subject to personal attack, dismissal and enquiry for wishing to work in a different way from her colleagues exemplifies this in a very dramatic way (Savage, 1992).

The latent conflict between these interests became more visible as soon as there was any pressure for change through community action and it became clear that we needed to develop an analysis and a strategy to deal with this in practice.

The role of conflict in any strategy of social change has long been at the centre of strenuous debates within community work,

'The meaning of social conflict and its merits and liabilities in community action has been one of the major conceptual and practice issues that distinguishes the different schools of thought in community action.'

(Gilbert and Specht 1975)

The different schools of thought on this subject broadly reflect the different ideological perspectives of consensus, pluralist and conflict explanations of society. Across this spectrum there have been those such as William and Loureide Biddle, working in America in the 1960's, who from a conservative/religious position recognised different interests in society but believed that these could be mediated through community action to achieve consensus and unity (Biddle 1965). At the other end of the spectrum there have been writers and activists such as Alinsky (1946) who saw people's organisations as essentially conflict groups by their very nature.

Marris and Rein, examining community action programmes in the USA in the 1960's, noted the way that the term community organisation was used to cover a myriad of activities under the same heading, each of which had different values and purposes.

'Community organisation could be interpreted with a very different emphasis, according to the standpoint of the organiser. It could be used to encourage the residents of a neighbourhood to come to terms with the demands of a wider society, or conversely to force the institutions of that society to adapt more sympathetically to the special needs of a neighbourhood. Or it could be seen as a form of therapy, to treat apathy and social disorganisation. And it might take an individual bias – promoting the social mobility of potential leaders, championing causes of personal injustice – or a communal bias more concerned with the neighbourhood as a mutually supportive community.'

(Marris and Rein 1967)

Certainly the initial impetus behind the Pilton project and probably the views of the funding agencies demonstrated a more consensus position which assumed that if a link was made between the community and primary health care, this would improve the health status of people living in a 'deprived area'. The emphasis was on co-operation and dialogue – that it was primarily a matter of communication or better take up of existing health services. It was assumed that at some level there should be a harmony of interests. As the case studies demonstrate, this position proved untenable in many instances. Bryant provides a reminder of the different interests that are at stake in these interchanges.

'Just as in industrial relations it is naive to speak of a harmony of interests between employers and employees, so it is equally simple-minded to assume, in the field of community relations, a natural consensus of interests between, for example, council tenants and housing authorities, privately rented tenants and their landlords.....community action merely makes explicit the tensions and inequalities which may exist in various situations.'

(Bryant, 1972)

The experience of the Pilton project was not unique. As other projects developed throughout the UK, the tensions experienced were replicated in a number of projects which had been established within a medical setting. For example in a paper prepared for the Roots and Branches Winter School, the authors conclude with a section on sharing power.

'there is an unwillingness amongst professional groups to explore ways of breaking down professional barriers between the professional and patient/client and to share their knowledge and skills and ultimately, their power. This is especially the case in the NHS. Such professional

attitudes fly in the face of community development which focuses on working with disadvantaged people to develop ways in which they can gain power over their lives. The potential conflict between professional/NHS and community interests needs to be acknowledged if there is to be a realistic commitment to promoting community development within a statutory setting. In Salford, the job descriptions of the workers contain a clause recognising the potential for conflict stating that in such a situation the worker's responsibilities lie with the community rather than the Health Authority.'

(Jayneand Youd 1990)

The potential and the difficulties for both collaboration and for conflict between medical and community development perspectives in relation to health were brought into sharper focus during this pilot phase.

The Second Phase: Strengthening the Community Voice

It became clear from the early work described above, that the concerns of one small group such as the tranquillisers support group or local pensioner groups, would need support from a stronger base or a wider network if they were to be taken more seriously by service providers. The new aims for this phase reflected this change of thinking. These were:

– **to encourage a climate for the articulation of health related needs by the community**

– **to establish within the designated community a means for initiating and maintaining a participatory model of health promotion which will involve an active dialogue between community groups and between different professional groups in health, social and educational services.**

There was now emphasis on 'participatory structures' and an 'active dialogue' and this model was to be evaluated in terms of process and outcomes. The intentions were to strengthen the community voice by developing wider networks of common concerns and interests, which could be shared and channelled into co-ordinated action through single umbrella organisations and where appropriate, to form alliances with local professionals in order to present a stronger case.

The three case studies which follow attempt to provide an analysis of the effectiveness and the limitations of different forms of action which developed.

Case Study 1: The Chiropody Campaign 'Feet First'

The development of the Pilton Elderly Forum has been described in the previous chapter. The local chiropody services came up as one of the first major issues in the Forum. A chiropody clinic was provided in the local community centre but only for one session a month – on the second Tuesday of the month. Appointments had to be made by phoning on this particular day and the chiropodist who was there treating feet had to answer the phone to deal with the appointments as well. People had difficulty remembering which Tuesday it was and even the day was sometimes changed. There was a long waiting time for appointments and even longer for home visits. This poor service had a direct impact on elderly people who not only had to suffer pain and discomfort for long periods, but it reduced their mobility which in turn affected their social contacts and independence.

There was support for the campaign from local health professionals, the community health services manager who wished to improve the service, voluntary organisations, from local people, the local press who were sympathetic to the issue and liked seeing elderly people in action and of course the wide membership of the Pilton Elderly Forum (P.E.F.). At that time the Forum was serviced by the Health Project, which took minutes or had them typed and circulated and paid for the mailing. Forum business could be done on our phone and we supported various tasks identified by Forum members.

The obstacles to change at that time seemed to be a lack of concern by the Health Board and a chiropody service which did not seem to see any need to improve the service.

The relationship between different responses to particular issues has been identified by a number of writers. The typology developed by Warren (1969) describes three possibilities which require different modes of intervention.

Nature of the Issue	Mode of Intervention
Issue consensus where there is a high possibility of agreement between the people wanting change and those who could implement it	Collaborative e.g. problem solving, persuasion, education
Issue difference where there are differences between the two parties but the possibility of agreement exist	Campaigns, bargaining, negotiation, mild pressure
Issue dissensus where there is no agreement between the parties	Conflict, confrontation, disruptive tactics

In the Chiropody Campaign there was a high degree of consensus between an alliance of local people, local health professionals and the health services manager, and the local health council. There was also media and public support for an issue which clearly affected elderly people. The initial strategy in the campaign concentrated on persuasion by writing letters and holding public meetings. These bore no results but the resistance seemed to be from the area chiropodist and bureaucratic inertia rather than powerfully held opinions or widespread professional attitudes. Although the local health council had made various representations to the Health Board, the effects of this poorly run service on the elderly had not been forcibly drawn to their attention in a more concerted way and the Board had not bothered to investigate this issue.

The next tactic, was therefore, to exert some mild pressure and some education. The health project suggested a survey of local health professionals' views, particularly those who dealt with the elderly such as district nurses, GPs, health visitors and occupational therapists. Through the Forum, many of them had already individually expressed their dissatisfaction with the service and the strategy was to weld this support together into a more powerful collective stance. The Forum also decided to organise a petition from the local area, coupled with publicity. The health project also linked with the local arts worker who then worked with a group of pensioners to construct a large six feet high foot which was displayed in the local shopping centre, sporting the slogan – 'Cut our Nails not our Services!' Lastly the campaign was widened in collaboration with the Edinburgh Health Council, to include other areas in Lothian.

Elderly people in the area took to the campaign with relish! The chiropody clinic was eventually provided on a weekly basis and management changes within the chiropody service enabled them to attend to more home visits and the waiting list dropped. This example shows that community action can be very effective, even if there is issue difference between those who use the service and those who provide it, if the local organisation is well grounded and supported and alliances can be forged with some professional groups and agencies in order to exert mild pressure on the service providers.

However, despite some small successes in overcoming resistance to improvements or changes, we became aware of how fragile these new developments were – how easy it was for 'the sand to fill in the hole'. New developments which contained any challenge to the status quo or required even a slight change of power relationships were difficult to sustain. The next case study illustrates this process.

Case Study 2: Listening Ear, Mental Health Forum

A local Mental Health Forum was developed on rather similar lines to the Elderly Forum although the initial meetings were less straightforward as there were fewer established groups and organisations dealing with mental health issues in the area. The few that existed had been developed by the health project. In a

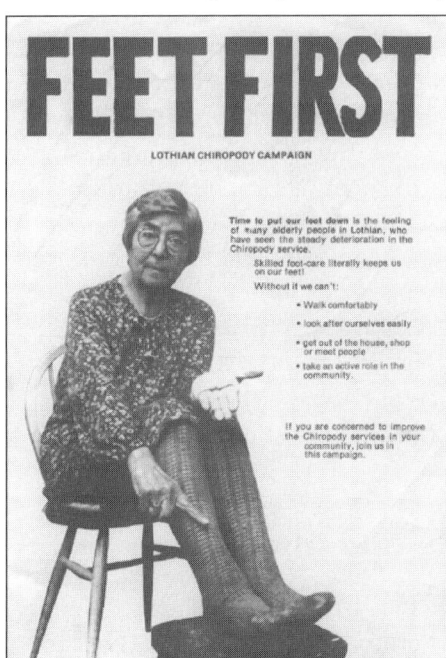

'Feet First' campaign flier.

large mixed meeting it was hard for local people who had experienced a loss of confidence through the experience of mental ill health to voice their opinions. At some of the initial exploratory meetings with local mental health professionals it was apparent that they had a very strong need to meet with each other for support and communication. This was the basis of some difference of opinion at first. Many professionals assumed that a mental health forum would consist largely of other professionals working in the area. This was not unsurprising as this is often the conventional model for such groupings and was happening in other areas. This is not to suggest that professional forums are invalid but simply that our particular concern was in developing opportunities for local people to have their say.

An initial meeting between local people and professionals was very cautious and there was some hesitation about the way forward. The Health project took the initiative in organising the next series of meetings in the community. Again the model was to ensure that there was a majority of local people and that they took the lead in identifying issues. Once this was observed the Mental Health Forum became very quickly established and was well supported by local people, who decided on its name – The Listening Ear, Pilton Mental Health Forum.

Parasuicide and After Care

The first important issue raised at the Listening Ear Forum was the lack of after-care for people who had been discharged from hospital after attempting suicide (parasuicide). In Edinburgh, at that time, people were admitted to one specific ward in the Royal Infirmary, the main teaching hospital. This was a medical ward and not part of the community psychiatric services.

At Forum meetings people described how they felt they had been 'washed out and turned out'. Their physical needs had been attended to – poisonous substances were removed and physical injuries patched up but their emotional needs were ignored. They also felt that they were not merely ignored but treated with some disdain and that some procedures were deliberately punitive. A nurse participant confirmed this, saying that it was not uncommon for people who had attempted suicide to be seen as a nuisance as against other patients who were more 'worthy' and that larger tubes than necessary were sometime used to pump stomachs 'so they wouldn't try it again'. One man described how he had been told he should go home and when he got outside the hospital he was overcome with despair and confusion. He had been through this tremendous crisis and was now back out on the street with no suggestion of any help, and with no bus fare even to get home. He had to walk across town back to his home and the same situation which had led to his crisis. (Video: After You Leave the Surgery, 1988). Having a forum controlled by local people enabled crucial issues like this to be aired more fully and it was tackled in a variety of ways.

Dialogue, Education and Persuasion

The Forum decided to talk with one of the consultants on the ward in the Royal Infirmary about parasuicide and after care. There was some anxiety about entering 'their' territory and eventually it was decided that two Forum members would go, the health project worker and a local resident. During the meeting with the consultant the discussion turned to the type of help and support that could be made available when people were about to be discharged from hospital. The consultant felt that in his experience this was not a priority as he had found people did not want to talk after a suicide bid, that the experience had somehow given them a new perspective on life and they often just wanted to get out of hospital and get on with things. Despite suggestions that this might not always be the case, the conversation stuck at this point as there seemed no meeting of minds.

The creation of a more positive dialogue was made possible by the counter-experience of the local resident who had been in this ward some years earlier. She was able to say with some authority that, although it had not been easy to talk in hospital because she was still in a state of shock, as soon as she had been discharged and begun trying to cope back home, it would have been extremely helpful to have had someone to talk to about what had happened. This information changed the nature of the discussion. The consultant could not argue with this real experience put before him and seemed to listen more attentively. There was also the element of surprise as though he had assumed the two members from the Forum were both professional workers and would not be bringing their personal experience of the service with them. His reaction was immediately more positive and he began to shift his opinion. He agreed to consider how such links could be made and to talk about this to his staff. He later became supportive of the small changes that were made within this ward.

This example demonstrates the value and power of equal dialogue and the importance of creating opportunities for it to happen.

Professional Alliances

The strong card the Mental Health Forum held in this issue was the alliance with the community psychiatric nurses (CPN's). They were also concerned about the lack of after care and also wanted to develop their work to cover this ward and were therefore willing to add their professional muscle in supporting the community demand for connections and networks of support to be set up between the ward and the community, because the outcome would complement their professional concerns. Staff from the ward – doctors, nurses and social workers, were invited to a special meeting to discuss the matter further and to draw up a proposal. For many of these staff it was probably the first time they had had such a discussion in a forum where there was a majority of lay people and in this case with a good many of them ex-patients of that ward. Because it was on their home ground, local people were more able to speak out and support one another. The dialogue and the balance of power felt more equal and a constructive and useful discussion ensued.

Discussion

There were two outcomes of this work. Firstly, a leaflet, designed and written by Forum members, was produced detailing three or four local groups who would be available to provide a 'Listening Ear' as well as details of local psychiatric services. Secondly it was arranged that the local psychiatric nurse would go into the ward on a weekly basis and if there were any people from the local area he would make contact with them, tell them what was available and leave them with a leaflet. Leaflets about other agencies in other areas were also collected and put into the ward.

This case study illustrates some of the possible tensions involved in 'intersectoral collaboration'. If the Mental Health Forum had been professionally dominated it would have expressed different set of concerns, but might have had more clout and been taken more seriously. However it may not have been as successful in expressing the 'community voice', in involving so many local people in its organisation or creating opportunities for professionals to listen properly to the concerns of local people. The value of creating opportunities for a more equal dialogue to take place, not only individually (between members and the consultant) but on a collective basis (between the ward staff and the whole forum) should not be underestimated. It was not only important in terms of improving communications between providers and users of services so that services could be more effective but it also allowed people to take back some of their own power and exert more control over how services are provided. It was fulfilling the progressive spirit of Alma Ata:

'people have the right and the duty to participate individually and collectively in the planning and implementation of health services'

Case Study 3: The Clinic Users Group

This example expands on the issues outlined in the first section on primary health care when it was noted that responses from health professionals depended very much on how much change was involved. It shows that the way in which issues are perceived dictates the response by those who have the most power in the situation.

The West Pilton Clinic was a small friendly local clinic based in a rather shabby pre-fab building providing child health, dental and family planning services for the immediate area. A report on the work of this group gives an introduction to how the Clinic Users' Group began.

'About five years ago the West Pilton Clinic was in danger of closure. The fabric of the building had deteriorated and poor security made it an easy target for vandals. This made it a depressing environment for staff and clinic users alike and

eventually many staff refused to work from the premises. After this low point in the Clinic's history, the importance of a local clinic in the area was acknowledged by the Health Board and an improvement programme was carried out. The building was made more secure and was brightly repainted. This was a boost for staff morale and to build on this positive move, a Clinic Users Group was established'.

(Alexander K, Beagley, M 1988)

Initially this did not include any users of the service but after prompting from the health project, the first two parent users were invited onto this group by the health visitor who then changed jobs during this period, to work with the health project. It was agreed that she should remain a member of this group and Chair the meetings.

The health visitor's role in chairing the meetings as she moved jobs and joined the Health Project meant that she was familiar to both the parent representatives and to her previous colleagues and this helped provide the bridge we needed between the Health Project and the primary health care team.

The parent users brought a number of issues to the Clinic Users Group and also, to canvas broader opinion, carried out a survey of local women. The survey included questions about the use of the clinic and what people knew about the services provided there. The results of the survey showed that many local people were unaware of what services were available locally and that afternoon appointments for the baby clinic were hard for mothers with older children at nursery or school.

It is worth examining a few of the different issues and the responses by the clinic staff to them. These were outlined in a report produced by the parent users after being involved in the Clinic Users Group for a number of years.

It can be seen that some areas are more amenable to change than others. For example, the issue of a play area for children was eventually accepted as it had the support of nearly all staff and was a demand from users of the clinic but it was dealt with informally and not taken more seriously at this stage. It rested on the goodwill of the receptionists who kept an eye on the children, toys brought in by staff and local people and was not adequately resourced. The times of the clinics, which were shown by the parent users to be inconvenient for many women with older children were not changed and not even considered as an item for change. The times were convenient for doctors and that was it! Other issues which were amenable to change were getting names of professionals on the doors in the clinic and producing a leaflet about the clinic.

These different examples show the strengths and limitations of attempts at collaboration or co-operation over particular issues. They show how the way the issue is 'perceived' dictates the response. Brager and Specht have extended the typology developed by Warren which was outlined earlier, and this version helps to illustrate what was going on in this particular interaction.

When Goal Perceived as	Response is	Intervention
Mutually enhancing adjustments/ re-arrangements of resources	Consensus	Collaborative
Redistribution of resources	Difference	Campaign
Change in status/ relationships	Dissensus	Contest or disruption

This framework is useful in understanding the progress of different issues. So, for example, when no one stands to lose status or control and the changes are perceived to be a minor rearrangement of resources, such as allowing toys in the reception area, 'collaboration' is possible. If existing status relationships are challenged, as with parent users dictating times of clinics, the response is likely to be dissensus, and contest or disruption may be the only mode able to produce change. The other important element noted by Brager and Specht is that although there are many instances where there will be a commonality of interests and the potential for collaborative tactics:

'this is less often the case than the widespread use of collaborative tactics would suggest. Its use might best be explained as a consequence of the unequal power of service users in relation to officials. When the reach of the poor is modest, it is, by and large, because their less potent resources require less strident behaviours....

To collaborate because there are common interests – or because one has no other alternative – or to "appear" to collaborate for political advantage, is reasonable. But to prescribe collaborative means as preferential, if not exclusive, methods, as do many professionals, is another matter. It is, we suspect, making a virtue of necessity.'

(Brager, Specht, 1973)

This view is echoed by the parent users who also saw that despite some gains, their impact was limited and that they needed to develop a stronger 'voice'.

'The response within the Clinic Users Group to parents having a voice was mostly positive considering most of the members had not been involved in such a group before. We feel our voices would be heard more easily if we had a stronger group of parent users...

There is still a long way to go before a community voice is heard by all professionals in the area. Many are set in their ways and don't want to change the system to our way of thinking. We still don't agree on priorities.'

(Karen Alexander and Marilyn Beagley 1988)

Although this framework is useful for theorising about tactics, in practice these three models of interaction overlap and merge into one another, depending on the particular response, and how much leverage a group can muster. Theory poses collaboration and conflict models as alternative models but they are not always choices.

Collaboration and consensus are possible only when both parties have the power to negotiate.

'The starting point of a community action campaign is not whether consensus or conflict is the most appropriate strategy to adopt but rather from the issues at stake, the organisational strength of the community, the nature of the opposition, the degree of participation and the experience of local leadership. ....communities use all available strategies but, ultimately, are forced into confrontation because a conflict of interests between them and the authorities is inherent in their situation.'

(Jacobs, 1975)

People with little power can often only begin to create a stronger identity when engaged in a conflictual situation with more powerful groups and a large body of sociological theory argues that inter-group conflict is the norm rather than the exception and provides the necessary 'fuel' for social change (Labonte 1997). In fact a number of authors have concluded that rather than an either/or scenario, conflict can be seen as an aspect of collaboration. Collaboration usually requires a stage when less powerful groups establish their legitimacy through a challenge to more powerful groups and this potential challenge acts as a lever to sustain the joint venture on a more equal basis.

Conclusion

The possibilities for change and intervention are heavily influenced by how the issue is perceived, and how much adjustment to existing power relations has to take place. Inter-sectoral work has to move from a dependence on single sympathetic individuals to a change in practices, procedures and resources which actively support community involvement.

Most of the examples in this chapter focus on initiatives which met with varying degrees of resistance from within the health service in order to develop an analysis of the potential and the limitations of inter-sectoral collaboration as a strategy for change. There were of course many individual health professionals and health units such as the Royal Victoria Rehabilitation Unit who supported activities and actions in a variety of ways and with whom we worked very happily.

On the whole, collaboration with other workers, local organisations and city wide agencies was less problematic and the wide range of collaborative partnerships that were developed was a significant feature of the project's work providing a supportive, interdependent network that was highly valued.

References

Alinsky, S (1946)	Reveille for Radicals. University of Chicago Press
Biddle, W and Biddle, L J (1965)	The Community Development Process Holt. Rinehart and Winston, New York
Brager, G and Specht, H (1973)	A Perspective on Tactics, Community organising. Columbia University Press, New York
Bryant, R (1972)	Community Action, Br. Journal Social Work, Vol.2 No.2.
Cohen, J M and Uphoff, N T (1979)	See in Macdonald, J (1993), Primary Health Care: medicine in its place. Earthscan
Freire, P (1972)	Pedagogy of the Oppressed. Penguin, Harmondsworth
Gilbert, N and Specht, H (1975)	Socio-political coordinates of community action: conflict, political – integration and citizen influence in Sociology of Community Action, ed, Leonard,P, Sociological Review monograph, 21. University of Keele
Jacobs, S (1975)	Community Action in a Glasgow Clearance Area, in The Sociology of Community Action, ed, Leonard, P. University of Keele
Jayne, L and Youd, L (1990)	In or Out of the NHS? paper in 'Roots and Branches' papers from the OU/HEA 1990 Winter School on CD and Health Open University
Labonte, R (1997)	Community, Community Development and the forming of Authentic Partnerships in Community Organising and Community Building for Health, ed, Minkler, M. Rutgers University Press, New Brunswick, New Jersey and London
Marris, P and Rein, M (1967)	Dilemmas of Social Reform. Routledge Keagan Paul
Martin, C J, Platt, S D and Hunt, S M (1987)	Housing Conditions and Ill Health, BMJ, Vol.294, 2/5/87
Martin, C J (1989)	Researching the obvious and influencing the influentials, Local Government Policy Making ,Vol.16, pp 47-51

Rosenthal, H (1983)	Neighbourhood Health Projects: some new approaches to health and community work in parts of the UK, Community Development Journal, Vol.18 No.2, pp 120-31
Savage, W (1992)	A Savage Enquiry: Who Cauhols Childbirth? Virago
Smith, S J (1990)	Health Status and the Housing System, Soc. Sci. Med., Vol No.31 (7), pp 753-62

Pilton Health Project Reports/Videos

Jones, J (1986)	Royston/Wardieburn: Final Report
Alexander, K and Beagley, M (1988)	West Pilton Clinic Users Group: User participation in practice
(1998)	After you leave the Surgery
In the Clear (1984)	Video made by 'Video in Pilton' about the way the community in Pilton became involved in the Mass X-ray campaigns in the 1950's and how the trade union campaign to draw attention to housing conditions was side lined.

WEST PILTON CLINIC USERS GROUP

User Participation in Practice

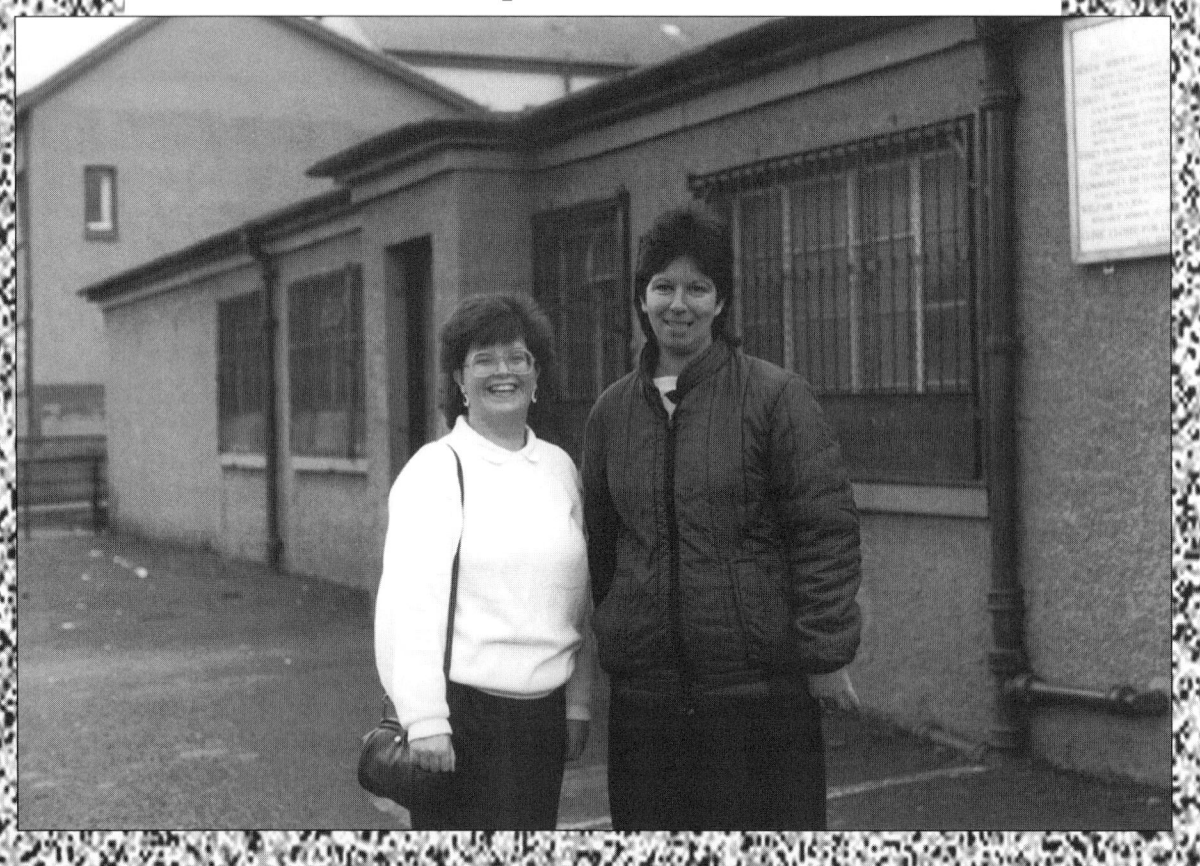

Community Control

Detail from Clinic Users Report.

Introduction

In the previous chapter the difficulty encountered when working for any kind of social change which challenged the status quo was likened to trying to plant trees in the desert. Nevertheless, as a result of the persistence of local people, the work of the health project and the support from some key officials within the local authority and the health service a number of 'trees' were eventually planted. Initiatives and services such as the Pilton Elderly Project, the Barrie Grubb Good Food Project, the Pilton Counselling Service and the PROP Stress Centre took root and flourished. Improved facilities in the local clinic and a return of a Minor Injury Unit at the local hospital were some of the more significant concrete achievements.

The development of local services such as these raises one of the other long standing debates within community work – the different emphasis and importance given to the 'process' and the 'product'. The redistributive function of community development in gaining resources and developing local services has usually been more easily supported by funders than the reality of 'community participation' and 'empowerment'. This is in part due to a lack of clarity about these concepts but it is also due to the advent of welfare pluralism, the business and managerial approach within the NHS and the development of Community Care. These have introduced a concentration on 'products' and 'services' and many health projects are being forced into unrealistic contracts which see the effectiveness of the work only in terms of providing services, and sometimes services which were previously provided by the state at a higher cost. The different philosophy behind the services developed through a community development approach can lead to different styles of working practice, a more inclusive management structure, and increased community access and involvement. It often seems as though the funders' interests are concentrated on how many people come through the doors and whether the service can be provided more cheaply. The potential for learning why and how services can be more effective and well used is lost. To gain the most from these developments there needs to be an understanding on behalf of funders, politicians and mainstream professional workers of how a 'product' or service is inextricably linked to an ongoing process of community development.

The services and initiatives listed above were a result of the community defining, demanding and creating more innovative, accessible or appropriate services and provided many benefits for local people. However as well as the undoubted benefit for the community in having access to these local services or projects, there were other equally important, although perhaps less visible gains from the process involved in achieving these.

Firstly, for the individuals involved in developing these or working in them, there was a gain in confidence, knowledge, skills and employment opportunities. Secondly they represented a not insignificant re-distribution of resources. Significant amounts of money were won for these health initiatives from the Urban Aid programme, from social work services, from charitable trusts, from the Scottish Office, from the local Pilton Partnership, which was part of the European Poverty programme, and from the Health Board. Thirdly, they represented a shift in power relations. People who had seen themselves as merely 'users' of services began to provide services and support for others. People's knowledge of mental health or providing healthy food was given equal value to that of other expertise and utilised through their employment in these initiatives. Local people developed skills in management and became management committee members or Directors of these separate autonomous projects.

Two American researchers (Cohen and Uphoff 1979) who examined a number of social development projects which claimed they were participatory drew out four types of participation:

a) people participating in setting the project up

b) people enjoying the benefits of the project

c) people evaluating the project

d) people making decisions about the project

They suggested that the first two were most common and that the last two, evaluating and making decisions about the project were the least common but the most significant in terms of people having more control.

Finally as well as seeing these concrete achievements and appreciating the importance of the process for individual participants, we began to appreciate the wider symbolic significance of such gains. Local people could see resources being developed, important services being fought for and retained through local community influence and action.

Community Control?

These developments represented different ways of organising services and drew on the knowledge and skills of local people, who had not been professionally trained in the health field. Although in many cases they did influence the professionals who had contact with them, we began to appreciate the subtle

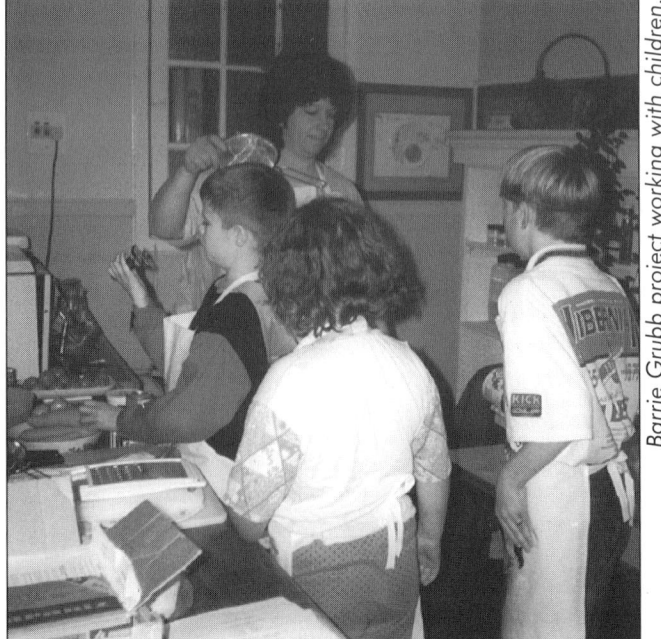

Barrie Grubb project working with children.

ways in which the status quo was maintained by existing dominant groups. We were beginning to identify the myriad ways in which the 'empowerment' process was thwarted.

This led us to try to ensure that these new resources and facilities were 'owned' by the community and that they had control over them. We also realised that unless this control was worked at and in some cases continually maintained and actively supported, the gains that had been won through community action could all to easily be diluted, co-opted, or even lost completely and the sand would fill in the hole again. The process is not straightforward. Following the progress of two initiatives described in the previous chapter demonstrates how assumptions and structures which dominate other types of services can lead even supportive professionals to undermine this type of development, sometimes without thinking.

Clinic Users Group

The local Pilton clinic in which the parent users had been so effective was planned for closure and this local service was to be provided in a large newly built clinic, a quarter of a mile away, which was to provide services for the whole of the north west of Edinburgh. The two parent users were asked to sit on the commissioning group for this new clinic. This seemed like a golden opportunity to extend the role of local people and they took up the offer with enthusiasm. They suggested a number of changes to the building to allow better access and insisted on a crèche facility. A crèche and crèche worker were accordingly provided – a positive addition much appreciated by local parents and comparatively rare in community health services. Once the building was completed they were then invited onto the larger management committee of the new clinic and continued to attend these meetings for almost another year. However, gradually their enthusiasm was worn down by this large committee. They felt that its membership was constantly changing, that it was hard to understand how and which decisions were being made and they felt that there was not the same commitment to hearing the user voice. If their views differed, they were challenged about how representative their views were (despite the fact that very few of the professionals were there in a representative capacity). They eventually decided to withdraw from the committee.

On reflection, although some minor successes were achieved and the parent users gained a lot in knowledge and confidence, what we had failed to do was to build more community support for their isolated position on this large committee. After they left, the health project made an attempt to push for user representation but after conducting a survey of users of the clinic we also realised that the structure itself mitigated against community involvement. This large clinic covered the north west sector of Edinburgh, offered a variety of specialist services and included over fifty different staff – there were many different 'communities' it was serving. Trying to build a participatory structure from one local neighbourhood was impossible.

Listening Ear Mental Health Forum

A second example of how small gains can be eroded is that of the initiatives outlined in the last chapter by the Listening Ear Mental Health Forum to offer support for people who had attempted suicide. The Forum had persuaded the hospital to let CPN's visit patients and to distribute a leaflet outlining the range of local support that was available to them once they were discharged. This worked well for about nine months or so but then it began to break down. There were a number of reasons for this:

- **staff changes on the ward meant that some of the key people who had initially agreed the plan had moved on and had not passed on the information to newcomers. Presumably it had low priority.**
- **a new consultant was appointed and they were not so keen on the CPN coming in so regularly and it became difficult for him to continue.**
- **the CPN's workload was also building up in the community.**

Interestingly, none of these professional staff had thought to inform the Forum of these changes which were to eventually jeopardise the initiative. If there had been prior warning, the Forum would have been able to organise to meet the new staff and re-state the need for such a network. It was apparent that the Listening Ear Forum was not seen as an integral part of their professional network but something marginal and that the concerns about support identified by local people had not been taken on board seriously.

This exposed our naivity in relying on individual goodwill. It showed us that changes to initiatives, however small, need to be formally incorporated at senior management level if they are to survive, so that they become part of policy not just a matter of goodwill or the positive attitude of individual staff.

Using methods and developing structures which developed and maintained community influence over the longer term meant in practice, for example, that the management committee of the Pilton Elderly Project, which had been initiated by the Pilton Elderly Forum described earlier, contained a majority of elderly people and that they formed the majority in important working groups such as interviewing panels.

The conventional way of providing services for people are built on certain assumptions and professional attitudes. The points raised in earlier sections about how hard it is for individual professionals to act differently from their colleagues has a bearing on new innovative schemes. Any new initiative which might wish to see different relationships develop or approach an issue from a non-traditional stance is extremely fragile. In the early stages, they need some protection so they do not get dismissed or discounted or alternatively co-opted by the existing mainstream services. This is an enduring tension in any work which is about change. Although there is a desire to influence the way mainstream services are provided, once a new idea catches on, control is lost and often the essential ingredients diluted.

The case study of the Middle House Stress Centre, which follows, illustrates some of the methods adopted in the development of the centre which tried to ensure that community control was built into the fabric of the place.

Case Study: The Middle House Stress Centre

For people who have experienced extremes of vulnerability, loss of confidence and powerlessness, the idea of initiating action and having some control over events seems daunting. The issues are much sharper and the obstacles seem bigger. The overall development of the Stress Centre, a user led centre for people experiencing stress and other mental health problems, has already been described in an earlier chapter and so this section focuses specifically on the task of enabling people to gain and maintain control over the running of the Centre.

Who is setting the agenda?

Determining community control over such a centre needs to be built into the bricks of the place. The ideas for the centre came from work with members of the tranquillisers support group during a Review Day and built on people's experience of the psychiatric services.

Membership and Relationships

Different types of relationships were wanted in the centre, relationships which were more equal and which both valued the experience and knowledge gained from living with mental health problems as well as professional knowledge. This value needed to be expressed as a concrete reality, in opportunities for equal employment. The employment of the two women who had been running the tranquillisers group, as lay mental health workers, utilised and acknowledged their expertise in working in the community, dealing with tranquillisers, and running groups as well as their personal qualities of empathy and respect for people.

There was a long debate about what to call people who came to the centre. Terms such as 'users' were rejected, as conveying a more passive taking of what was offered, and 'clients', 'consumers' or 'patients' as only describing one aspect of a relationship. The Greek root of the word client is 'one who is controlled'. The decision to call people who came to the centre, 'members' was significant in that it conveyed more democratic aspirations and a more active role, one which allowed people to move from 'disadvantaged object' to active subject. A role for people to contribute as well as take and to participate in the planning and running of the centre.

Members' Meetings

After the Middle House Centre had been running for about nine months, there were over thirty members. More decisions had to be taken. Issues of confidentiality, how to use the space, what sessions were wanted, all had to be dealt with and so the idea of Members Meetings was introduced. People were unused to and perhaps slightly apprehensive of 'meetings'. Their experiences had often been negative – meetings had been situations when their treatment had been decided, usually occasions when they felt anxious or powerless and so they began fairly informally. The health project worker chaired them and wrote up notes, ensuring that each member's comments were included. These were typed up and sent to members' homes. A superficial appraisal might see this as overly formal or trying to mimic larger hierarchical structures, but the intentions were quite different. Some members remarked that this was the first mail they had received for some time. People who are actively engaged in the world, whom others want to communicate with, receive mail. It's some kind of public acknowledgement that you exist and that you are important. These small details are important in practice – having your comments noted, made concrete and shared is acknowledging your worth.

Gradually members took on the role of chairing the meetings, taking notes and typing them up. Initially people who seemed to be a bit more confident were asked but as the meetings became more active and part of the Centre's life, elections were held as more people wanted to be involved in this way.

In the beginning the Members Meeting decided on practical things such as particular sessions they wanted to see in the programme and planned outings. As these suggestions were taken up people's confidence in things happening because they had suggested them or brought their own ideas forward, grew and an examination of the notes over time shows a steady confidence in tackling difficult areas such as the rights and needs of individuals versus the needs of the whole group. For example, space for smokers and non-smokers, whether someone could join a closed group after it had begun. This illustrates the importance of people seeing the concrete and visible effects of their contributions and suggestions, encouraging a sense of their personal effectiveness.

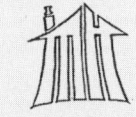

Summer in the Middle House Stress Centre

WHAT'S ON WHAT'S ON WHAT'S ON WHAT'S ON

Tuesdays

```
9.30–11.00am    Discussion   Individual time
1.30–3.00pm     Arts and Crafts
```

Thursdays

```
10.00–12.00     Drop in
11.00–12.00     Relaxation
12.30–1.30pm    Communal lunch
2.00  3.30pm    Building Confidence
```

You can phone the house on Tuesdays and Thursdays **Tel. 552 0404**

It was also important for people to control the boundaries of their own centre. In psychiatric hospital there was no say over who came in to see them, who knew about them or what activities they wanted to attend. There was an agreement that no private notes on people would be kept, only basic details of name, address and how and when they came to the Centre. Notice of people wanting to visit would be brought to the monthly members meeting and people would have the right of veto if they didn't wish someone to visit; that these visits should be restricted to once a month and that members would be the people to show them round. The right of veto was only used once but it was important for people to see that they did have this control and that workers were serious about supporting this decision.

The Centre flourished and grew and needed to begin to develop structures which would support its independence from the parent health project. It needed to develop some management structures and people's experience of being involved in the Members Meeting was a useful preparation for taking part in the Management Committee.

The members decided which professionals should join the management committee and through the constitution, that members should always be in the majority. This process was not an attempt to be crudely anti-authority or to suggest that professional skill was not important. There was respect for expertise but on the basis of a more equal dialogue. People wanted to learn from or be helped by professional skills but they did not want to be disempowered in the process.

These principles were carried forward as the Management Committee made an application for Urban Aid funding for a purpose built Stress Centre, to be called Pilton Reach Out Project (P.R.O.P.). The members worked with a community architect to design and shape their new building. Another member became employed as a worker and the Centre eventually became a local resource operating from its own building, with its own funding and management structure. An evaluation of the Middle House Stress Centre showed that members recognised the value of this.

'In hospital, even the trainee nurses think – I'm in authority. The Stress Centre workers are one of us, there's no class distinction. There are no records.'

'I was pushed from pillar to post until I found this place and then they gave me the confidence now to stand up and just put the brakes on and say I will not be pushed from pillar to post. I'm a person, a human being and I'm going to be heard.'

Discussion

Changes of this nature challenge the status quo of social and political relationships. The 'individual pathology' model, which underpins many professional approaches within the welfare state, sees the professional role as ameliorating individual dysfunction. We can see this in the biological or physical sphere where illness is treated; within the province of social services where support is given to 'dysfunctional' families; or within the remit of health education where people are persuaded to change their unhealthy behaviours. The emphasis within this model is on illness or inadequacies rather than on strengths or wider economic or political structures. Even utilising a more liberal humanitarian ideology which sees people's behaviour in terms of external influences constructs a model of the victim of circumstances even if the 'victim' is not blamed. The person is still seen as passive rather than active, the object of services, not the subject. The Freirian concept of people being seen and treated as subjects who know and act, rather than objects which are known and acted upon, had a large influence on the way the project developed and is explored more fully in a later chapter (Freire, 1972).

In the early 1970's, Richard Bryant, drawing from contemporary American experience also reflected on the way in which this idea challenges existing assumptions:

'groups and individuals, who previously have been defined as "passive" or "apathetic", may emerge through an involvement in community action as being active and organised, challenging conventional wisdoms and the competence of established institutions and official personnel.'

(Bryant 1972)

Changing the usual power relationships between professionals and lay people or between workers and members within such a Centre is complicated and stressful at times. This fact needs to be openly acknowledged by both parties and constantly worked with, reflected upon, supported and struggled with.

If people are experiencing mental ill-health, there will be times when they may not attend meetings but there are many occasions when professional members of management committees do not turn up or miss meetings. Years of being treated as stupid and worthless do not disappear overnight and the confidence required to take an active part in decision making have to be gradually acquired. There is bound to be a tension between the task and the process. The process of 'empowerment' in this situation needs active support and the time needed for training or developing alternative structures can compete with the more immediate task of running a centre or a service, for example. Here again the process and the product compete in a market economy which fragments the humanitarian and social from the consumer product. Funders, whether the health service or the local authority, have developed a narrow view of service provision, measured against a traditional view of what for example a 'day centre' should consist of – so many people in and so many out and how many sessions and how many staff needed to manage this 'business'. An initiative such as the Stress Centre certainly runs a highly efficient preventative service for people on a daily basis but it also runs an empowerment programme that is less visible and less easy to quantify than traditional work. If we are serious about increasing people's control over local services then both the tasks and the process need to be acknowledged and adequately resourced.

In the intervening years this principle of local control has been challenged by professionals in a number of the projects established by the health project. Towards the end of the 1990's as funding became more critical and community care influences the way services are being purchased a number of the projects described in this book are having to wrestle with this issue of co-option and local control.

Gaining resources also signals some recognition of a new or creative way of working but these often have to be fought for with some tenacity! After years of helping to develop a number of different food co-ops, we became frustrated that the hard work that was involved always had to be seen in a voluntary capacity. Middle class people do not have to devote their free time and energy a couple of days a week to ensure access to reasonably priced fresh fruit and vegetables. In 1993, the Scottish Office published a summary of 'The Scottish Diet' as part of their review of Scotland's health. This detailed the poor diets of low income groups and suggested that there needed to be an increase in the consumption of fresh fruit and vegetables but did not indicate where resources should come from to enable this to happen. We contacted the Scottish Office and said that we were trying to sustain an initiative, 'Barrie Grubb', which made fresh fruit and vegetables available, accessible and affordable to people on a low income and were there any resources that would be following the report? After being passed around a number of departments, we finally spoke to one official who was extremely doubtful that they could fund any such initiative. However, we sent him details of the Barrie Grubb Project and a week later, to our surprise saw that there was a reference to it from a Scottish Office spokesman in a press article about the Scottish Diet Report.

This was a useful lever to persuade this official to come down to the project and see what we were trying to do. Two months later we received funding to enable us to begin to pay some part-time staff to run the project. This was never quite enough but it enabled the project to develop its work, to create a precedent for food co-op workers to be paid, and more importantly to remind civil servants that policy changes require resource changes.

Concrete and visible achievements are important. Developing services and employment opportunities, particularly for more marginalised groups is an aspect of resource redistribution. There are also undoubted benefits for the individuals and groups most centrally involved in terms of personal, social or educational opportunities. However, gaining new services for the community or developing alternative, community controlled services has a wider significance. The whole process of defining, demanding and creating services which meet local needs defined by people themselves and which encourage more equitable relationships is a form of community action which has its own 'visibility'. It provides a day to day demonstration of growing confidence, self-respect and capability not only for those involved but as inspiration and encouragement to the wider community.

Although the numbers of people engaged in these community action initiatives is relatively small, perhaps their symbolic significance has been underestimated. Both the desire for, and possibility of, positive change, have to occur in the hearts and minds of people and particularly in people who have been made to feel powerless for much of their lives. Their experience of education and life may have taught them a number of harsh lessons; not to hope for much, not to challenge dominant interests, to shut up and keep quiet, not to expect 'too much'. Seeing things happen, seeing new resources being developed by other residents can give some optimism, can encourage more people to get involved and this whole process releases new energy. We need, however, to be watchful of attempts to colonise community initiatives in ways which reduce or eliminate the challenge they present.

For example, although the parent users in the Clinic Users Group had had an impact on the plans for the new clinic and its provision of childcare, their withdrawal from the committee, meant that these improvements are now just seen as part of the clinic, albeit a good model for other services, but not as a continuing symbol of the advantages of community involvement in the planning and delivery of services.

City's nurse-led minor injuries clinic given new lease of life

Herald and Post, 14 November 1996.

By BRIAN FERGUSON

A UNIQUE minor injuries clinic at the Western General Hospital will continue to get funding following the completion of the two-year pilot project.

Lothian Health paid £652,000 for the setting up of the walk-in clinic run primarily by nurses, in the hospital's main outpatients department, in November 1994.

More than 20,000 patients have been treated there since then and the pioneering clinic had won plaudits in national healthcare awards.

It was a runner-up in the prestigious Golden Helix Award this year and was highly commended in the Nursing Times 3M competition in November 1995.

Nurses at the clinic, which is open every day of the year, offer treatment for a wide range of minor injuries, including minor fractures, sprains, cuts, bites, minor burns and scalds.

A recent independent audit showed that more than 95 per cent of patients are happy with the care they received in the clinic - the only one of its kind in Scotland.

Carol Crowther, outpatient services manager for the Western General Hospitals NHS Trust, said: "Staff are delighted with the announcement of continued funding.

"The service has demonstrated clearly that it is answering a local need and many thousands of patients are happy with the prompt and expert nursing treatment and advice they are receiving."

Lothian Health's general manager, Trevor Jones, said: "There is no doubt that this clinic is meeting a real need in the communities that it serves, which is why we are continuing to fund it."

The wider community was initially very much aware of the gains made by the Western General Action Group in pushing for the local minor injuries service to be re-instated and in helping the hospital to consider a nurse practitioner-led model. However, as the newspaper cutting shows, a few years later, this extremely successful minor injury service is promoted by the hospital as one of its own achievements and the effort and commitment put in over four years by local people receives no mention.

The development of an innovative service such as the Stress Centre was possible because it built on the skills, knowledge, and understanding that members had about mental health and human relationships. It has value as an innovative, alternative model to psychiatric care, as a local resource developed and run by local people through their own efforts and continues to provide a much needed and highly respected service for the local area. It has influenced and inspired other communities to set up similar centres but it still remains a marginal project with an insecure financial future.

Conclusion

This chapter has tried to document attempts to learn from practice and be more conscious of the different tensions involved in concepts such as incorporation and community control. There will always be a tension between the mainstream and the community and this should not be viewed as negative but as part of the democratic push and pull. Community action which leads to concrete gains in terms of improved services, a respectful relationships between professional and lay knowledge, and increased resources has a value both for the community, for the individuals who have achieved this and holds symbolic significance for others in seeing that change is possible through their own action.

"It is only in the shared belief and insistence that there are practical alternatives that the balance of forces and chances begins to alter. Once the inevitabilities are challenged, we begin gathering our resources for a journey of hope."

(Williams, 1983)

References

Cohen, J M and Uphoff, N T (1977)	Rural Development Participation: Concepts and Measures for Project Design, Implementation and Evaluation. Cornell University
Freire, P (1973)	Education for Critical Consciousness. Seabury Press, New York
Bryant, R (1972)	Community Action, British Journal of Social Work, Vol.2 No.2
Williams, R (1983)	Towards 2000, Penguin, Harmondswaith

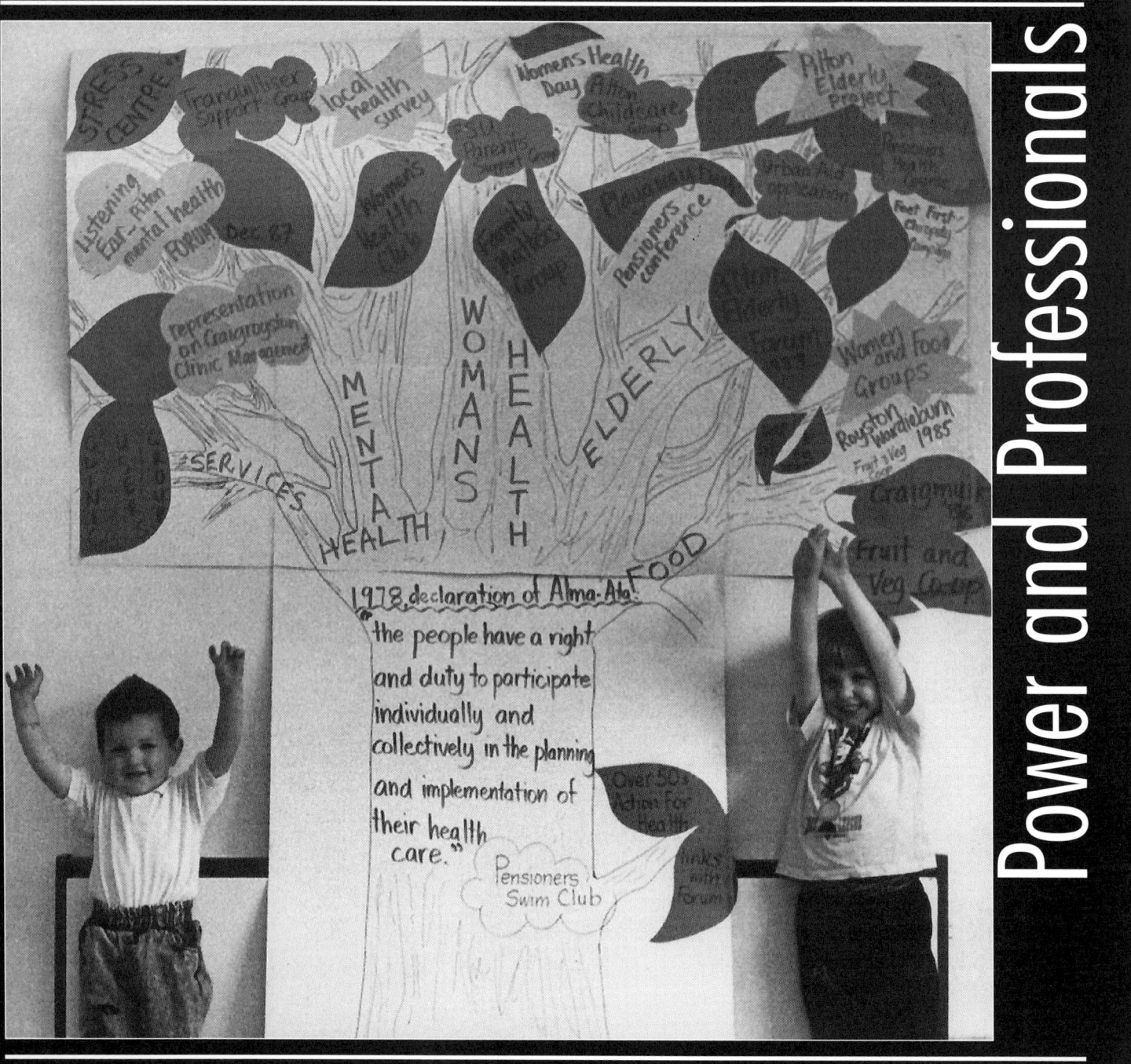

The project 'Tree' with the Alma-Ata Declaration at the centre.

Power and Professionals

Introduction

In the previous chapter, some of the obstacles which resisted change were examined. Some of these were obvious or more 'visible' and some were much more subtle and complex. The totality of this experience gradually revealed the way that power is exercised by particular interest groups and why reducing inequalities in health is so hard to achieve.

A critical perspective on power needs to include an understanding of what the exercise of power feels like to those who are affected by it. The French philosopher Foucault has emphasised that this is the appropriate way to understand power – to concentrate on the experiences of those who are subjected to this type of control, rather than on the mechanics of how it is exercised (Foucault 1986). The previous chapters illustrate some of the ways in which we tried to develop a deeper understanding of powerlessness – through listening to the experience of individuals, through attempts at community action, and observing and reflecting on this process. A sociological perspective is helpful in untangling the complex interdependence between the individual and social structures or as C. Wright Mills observed, to 'grasp history and biography, and the relations between the two, in society' (Wright Mills 1968).

In this chapter aspects of this process are examined in more detail, drawing on theories and ideas which help to explain our particular experience.

Perspectives on Power

Why is it appropriate and necessary to develop a perspective on power in community development and health work?

Firstly, the lack of power or control in people's lives has been identified as having a detrimental effect on health. In the 1970's and 1980's the psychosocial literature showed the importance of individuals' sense of control – the 'internal locus of control' on their health. In the early 1980's, research from the field of social psychology demonstrated the limitations of this individual model. A study looking at why some people remained well and others became ill, when subjected to similar stressful life events, identified a 'hardiness factor' or resistance to illness which included three key aspects. Firstly, the amount of control people felt they could exert over their lives; secondly whether they were committed or actively engaged in something that was meaningful for them; and thirdly whether they believed that change was an opportunity or a threat. The study concluded that people with this hardiness factor were less likely to become ill despite stressful events in their lives (Kobasa, Maddi and Kahn 1982). This identification of the importance of social cohesion or the relationship between an individual and their environment, begins to address issues of power and powerlessness and their effect on health.

In 1992, Wallerstein's comprehensive literature review examined the link between powerlessness and health, analysing studies undertaken in the health and social science literature covering areas such as social epidemiology, occupational health, stress, social support networks, community organising and social action. She concluded that powerlessness, or lack of control over destiny must be considered as a broad based risk factor for disease and ill-health. Attention was also drawn to the limitations of some of the social psychology literature in which control was defined within an individual dimension.

'One limitation of this research on individual control is that many who live in poverty or face discrimination may in fact have a an accurate appraisal of the extent of their control in the environment. Interventions which attempt to increase internal locus of control, without changing the environmental conditions, may increase frustration and lead to greater perceived powerlessness.'

(Wallerstein 1992)

Empowerment

The word 'empowerment' has become a vogue word. It is used liberally within health and welfare circles and like 'participation' or 'community' it can be used as a type of giftwrap to present a pleasing appearance whilst concealing more than it reveals.

In health promotion circles there has been a tension between those who maintain a focus on empowerment as individual change, as a technical 'skill' to be learnt, to improve self-confidence or self-esteem, to 'manage' stress or learn to cope, and those who advocate a move towards a social change model of empowerment (Adams and Pintus 1994). This reflects a similar ambiguity found in many major health policy documents and statements, including those from the World Health Organisation (WHO), which stress the importance of people having more control or 'empowerment' over the factors which affect their health. Once again, the focus is mainly on the subjective nature of powerlessness, reduced to individual behavioural problems which will be resolved through stress management courses or confidence building techniques and expounded without any acknowledgement of the political implications.

WHO documents such as the Alma Ata Declaration of 1978 and Health For All by the Year 2000 in 1986 have been criticised for their atheoretical pragmatism which obscures entrenched barriers to change and undermines the radical principles they espouse. (Farrant 1991, Navarro 1984)

'Although the central HFA (Health For All) focus on redressing inequalities would imply an emphasis on empowering oppressed and disadvantaged groups, the "community" and "the public" are frequently referred to as a homogenous whole, with little encouragement to systematically analyse power relations within and between communities. In so far as mention is made of the need to secure the participation of the disenfranchised, it is rarely acknowledged that participation involves conflict and confrontation as well as consensus and co-operation and, to be effective, would require a fundamental shift in the distribution of power.'

(Farrant 1991)

If community development is the process of working alongside people in identifying and articulating the issues which affect their health, an awareness of the processes which prevent these being articulated is a pre-requisite for effective practice. If community development is about encouraging people to act on the determinants of ill-health, both practitioners and local people need to also know about the obstacles involved in the social change process. Both aspects require an understanding of the way powerlessness is experienced by individuals and how power is exercised.

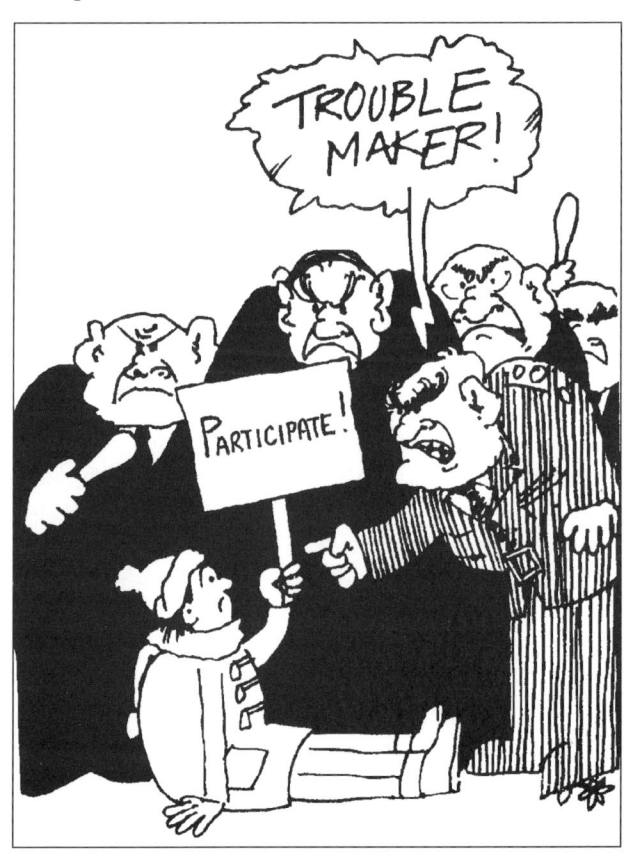

Theories about Power

Lukes' analysis of power and Alford's concept of structured interest groups within the health services are helpful in unravelling some of these complexities (Lukes 1974 Alford 1975).

Lukes' analysis opens up the concept of power in a way which allows us to understand both its subtleties and its pervasiveness. First of all he examines a **one-dimensional** or pluralist view of power. This view, characterised by the ideas of Max Weber and promoted by the work of Robert Dahl in the 1960's gained considerable influence amongst political scientists in America. It assumes that 'observable conflict' is the way we can understand the exercise of power by observing whose decisions are carried through when a conflict of views are expressed. This idea was developed by observing and recording whose decisions prevailed within key policy areas. The assumption that all struggles for power and control are played out by decision makers in the visible political arena was challenged by Lukes who recognised that many interests are not articulated at this level and in this form. He sees this kind of explanation as too limited, revealing only the tip of the iceberg.

The **two-dimensional** view of power, recognises interests which might not reach, or indeed are kept off, the official agenda of the dominant groups in society. This view sees the exercise of power as the ability of dominant groups to prevent conflict from even reaching the decision making arena by securing compliance through coercion, influence, authority, force and manipulation. In other words marginalising, circumventing, or ignoring less powerful groups or individuals' interests and 'mobilising bias' through organisational means.

This view, although recognising non-decision making as well as decision making as an exercise of power, still assumes that interests are consciously articulated and visible. Lukes' particular contribution is in taking a conceptual leap forward in forming a **three-dimensional** view of power. He makes the case that this close observation of behaviour and decision making does not take account of the most effective use of power which is to shape the way people think, and so prevent opposing views being articulated in the first place.

In this analysis he takes account of the way dominant ideologies influence, and are reflected in, the social systems and structures which in turn shape, and are shaped, by individuals – an analysis also shared by feminists writing in the same period,

'the prevailing social order stands as a great and resplendent hall of mirrors. It owns and occupies the world as it is and the world as it is seen and heard.'

(Rowbotham 1973)

In this way less powerful people's interests become defined by others within a system which ultimately works against them. For example, the focus on individual behaviour suggests that ill-health, experienced more widely by people on low income, is largely a result of people's bad habits such as smoking and eating unhealthy food rather than examining the effects of poverty or the distribution of income and wealth.

'when it was revealed once again that Glasgow had an appalling health record and had one of the highest premature death rates in Western Europe and was nominated heart disease capital of the world, it came as no surprise to us whatsoever. What did surprise us was that the blame was put on our diet and in particular our greasy fish suppers and general lifestyle. Not content to blame us for our appalling living conditions and poverty, officials and experts seemed determined to persecute us as well.'

(McCormack 1993)

Views which conflict with the dominant one are labelled 'subversive' and people who protest 'agitators' or 'trouble makers'. A variety of mechanisms are at work in society which help to maintain this dominant view in such a way that it becomes the only truth. The most insidious aspect of this is the way in which the least powerful groups begin to internalise the dominant view even when it acts against their own interests. They feel that their views are not acceptable, or that they are not capable enough to take part in civic affairs. If doctors make notes about your body or your mind, and do not let you know what is being planned for your treatment, you begin to feel that this is 'normal' and that to ask questions or demand more information is being 'difficult'. This three-dimensional view of power allow us to see how the least powerful begin to support their own oppression, so there does not have to be any 'observable' conflict or competing interest groups – people simply give up the struggle.

Marilyn Beagley who took a lead role in the Western General Action Group (often called trouble makers by health officials) expressed this very succinctly in a report she wrote for the project.

'It really annoys me that people sit back and let it happen. People inside the hospital are conditioned to accept these things and they have a loyalty to the doctors. People outwith the hospital, in the area – they are saying, you're wasting your time, the decision's been made and there is nothing you can do to stop it. I think people have been conditioned to listen to the "Big Yins" up there – not the wee folk.'

Robert Alford, a political scientist who studied New York City's health services for over twenty years identified interactions which maintained the status quo and repeatedly prevented change from occurring in the system. The interactions he observed occurred between three sets of 'structural interests'. His work has been interpreted in a way which helps us examine these different views of power within the context of the UK health services (Williamson 1988).

Interest Groups
Dominant – the 'professional monopolisers'
Challenging – the 'corporate rationalisers'
Repressed – the 'community interest'

The dominant interest group is described as those health care professionals who have a monopoly over the provision of their services. They are usually doctors but can include other health professionals who have gained control over their own conditions of working – a feature of a powerful professional group which we will return to later. These 'professional monopolisers' are numerically small but exert great influence, particularly as their definition of health still tends to dominate health policy and health provision. There is major support, politically, structurally and culturally for this dominant group.

The second major interest group identified by Alford is that of the 'corporate rationalisers' containing administrators, executives, managers, planners and those professionals whose main focus is on improving the efficiency and effectiveness of health services and whose guiding value base is the rational use of resources and 'value for money'. They try to challenge the dominant group by attempting to restrict their autonomous work practices and their use of resources. In the UK context, we can see how the introduction of general management within the NHS, and the creation of an internal market, has given more power to the 'corporate rationalisers'. Many commentators saw the desire to obtain some managerial control over doctors as the principal objective behind the Griffiths Report in 1983 and the introduction of general management into the NHS which followed. The move by many doctors into management positions in the late 1980's illustrated the struggle for control which is still continuing as the NHS continues to be re-structured. In the battle between these two interest groups, the third group's interests are even more invisible.

The interests of the third group, the 'repressed' group, are those of the community. In the American context, Alford sees this group as consisting of the rural and urban poor who might just earn enough not to qualify for Medicaid and who need accessible, low cost health care. Their interests are not supported by any social or political institutions. Their interests are often not even articulated within the prevailing social order. Attempts at organisation are further hindered by the interplay of the other two groups. As in Lukes' theory of power, Alford is recognising that pluralistic explanations of competing interest groups holding different amounts of power are insufficient and develops a more radical view which suggests that different interests are structurally supported, or 'repressed', through the social, political, economic and cultural institutions within society. He identifies how other groups in society, outside the health service, accept by and large the validity of health professionals' power through a myriad of everyday interactions and practice. For example, an acceptance of the dominant role that the medical profession plays in planning and organising our health service – automatically given places on Health Boards, or government working groups – over and above other professional groups, or community representatives despite the limited role medicine has in improving our overall health. The two examples that follow will attempt to demonstrate how some of these structures and the way we operate within them, support the dominant interest group in the field of health.

The Sick Role

The first example looks at a common interaction – visiting the doctor when we are sick. It examines the way in which this interaction is part of the way in which power is both accorded to and accepted by, the medical profession.

The relationship between the medical profession and the public is built upon a web of anxieties we feel when we become 'ill'. We have many reactions to not being 'well' which are not purely about pain or suffering but about the meaning it holds for us. In medieval times, illness was often associated with some type of punishment for transgressing religious or cultural mores and remnants of this belief still filter their way into contemporary belief systems. Research in the area of lay concepts of health reveals that a major recurring theme is that of health and illness as moral constructs. Responsibility, blame, guilt, hypochondria and stoicism, for example, are just a few of the morally evaluative terms regularly used by people to describe their relationship to their own health. (Research Unit for Health and Behavioural Change, 1989).

Being ill also relieves us of our responsibilities. We can stay away from school or work, and we are not expected to carry out our usual roles. Parsons' concept of the 'sick role' explains why the need to regulate this withdrawal from social and occupational duties is recognised by most societies in the world. Without such regulation society would have difficulty functioning (Parsons 1951). He also observed that being sick gives us both rights and obligations. We can be excused from our social duties but we also have an obligation to seek and follow the advice of others and obey doctor's orders. In other words we have a duty to try to get better. Our sick status needs to be legitimated by those, such as the medical profession, who are seen to have the required knowledge, status and prestige. To be considered for the benefits which society has granted to the 'sick', various public bodies such as the DSS or the Housing Department require a sick line or certificate from a medical doctor. The doctor therefore has a very powerful role as gatekeeper to resources and legitimator of our illness, backed up and supported by ourselves as patients and various other institutions and professions. The ability of physicians to take away the responsibility for being ill, to take over and deal with the illness, is one explanation of the power they hold in society and in relation to individual patients. We can see how this role fulfils individual needs, supports society to function in a particular way and also how it establishes a set of power relationships. Some circumstances reduce the power of the patient even further.

Powerlessness and Mental Health

People faced with mental illness often feel particularly powerless. To have a confusing and frightening emotional state labelled as a particular illness must be an immense relief. To find there are people who claim expertise and familiarity with this frightening experience, to 'name' it and recognise it as significant through treatment or hospital admission is part of the complex social and cultural investment in the doctor/patient relationship. The importance of the whole process is the meaning it gives to the illness state. It is not the individual's fault but the result of an outside agent or 'disease' identified by an expert. This legitimation is so powerful that if a claim to illness is not regarded as legitimate by the medical profession, the individual may be subjected to moral scrutiny, judgement and pressure.

Some members of the Middle House Stress Centre, made a video based on their experience of the psychiatric services and one of the accounts in the video demonstrates this desperate need for help which is consequent on this legitimation.

'I was still ill, so I went back to my own doctor and he said "I can't understand why you're depressed" and so I went back to the Royal Edinburgh and the doctor there looked at my notes and says "what are you doing here again... we can't do anything for you, you've been discharged. What are you doing wasting my time?" I thought, God, even they have turned against me. ...and I was really upset, because I'd three bairns to look after and that.

How did that make you feel?

I felt, again, about that size (making a tiny space between finger and thumb) that I must be bad, that perhaps I was wasting their time ... but I tried to cope for 2 or 3 weeks or months ... and eventually I took an overdose.'

Video: 'After You leave the Surgery'

An appreciation of the powerful forces which can lead us to concur with the role of the doctor can help us understand the resulting tensions when the benefits of the 'sick role' conflict with the obligations which come with it. In the area of mental health, the patient is sometimes faced with an intolerable choice. The immediate relief or reassurance obtained through the legitimation of mental illness is often contingent upon a number of obligations which can create a state of powerlessness and passivity in the individual.

Firstly mental health patients usually have to give up their control over the situation and accept the authority of the doctor and the institution. Secondly they have to accept the diagnosis and treatment given. They may also have to endure the objectification process which views part of their identity or personality as 'not right' and in need of medical treatment, whether by drugs, ECT or psychological forms of treatment. Two more extracts from the video show people's experience of this process.

'For about two days they gave me these tranquillisers although I didn't know at the time what they were and I started getting the shakes. I couldn't lie still and my body was jumping all over the place and I was aware that something was happening in my body – as though it was trying to reject the rubbish they were giving me. I went up to the nurse and said could it be the pills they were giving me because I felt really terrible and really irritable. They says "No, no it's just the way you're feeling, the tablets will calm you down". But they weren't calming me down and they weren't helping me sleep so I refused to take them after that.. and they gave me a hard time after that, you know, they really treated me badly. If I needed someone to talk to they wouldn't talk to me because I wasn't co-operating with "the system" you might say.'

'you just feel as though you're taking up their time and that they've got the answers as to how they're going to treat you with this tablet and that tablet and ..you really want help – at the level you're at, ken.'

Video: 'After You Leave the Surgery'

Lastly there is the longer term consequence of being labelled as mentally ill and all that implies for the rest of your life, or certainly for a much longer term than the period of treatment.

The stigma of being labelled mentally ill has been recorded by many researchers and sociologists.

'stigma is by definition, ineradicable and irreversible: it is so closely connected with identity that even after the cause of the imputation of stigma has been removed and the societal reaction has been ostensibly re-directed, identity is formed by the fact of having been in a stigmatised role: the cured mental patient is not just another person, but an ex-mental patient. One's identity is permanently spoiled... A stigma furthermore, that interferes with normal interaction, for while people need not hold the "deviant" responsible for his stigma, they are nonetheless embarrassed, upset or even revolted by it.'

(Freidson, 1970)

The label influences others' perceptions and friends, neighbours and even close family members may become uneasy about communication or making connections because they themselves are influenced by the label which puts the mentally ill person into a different category – outside 'normal' social activity. Challenging or disagreeing with the label will not be taken at face value but somehow as part of the illness. The individual's power and autonomy is reduced and compounded by every stage in this process and it is little wonder that many people begin to internalise this view, seeing themselves as mad, bad or hopeless.

Labelling theory was highly influential during the 1960's and was concerned with both the way that people were labelled as deviant, when their conduct did not fit with other's expectations and about who does the labelling. Some identified psychiatrists (Scheff 1966) and others such as Goffman (1961) identified a complex of different actors – the family, the professionals and the 'total' institution. The significance of the relationship between those labelled and those doing the labelling also holds useful insights in terms of definition being an exercise of power. Horwitz (1983) found that women were more likely to be labelled than men in lay networks and also that the greater the personal gap in terms of class, race, culture and gender between labellers and the potentially labelled, the greater the chance of being so defined and of the label being more devaluing.

Other theoretical positions have taken an even broader sweep in asserting that all deviance from the norm is socially constructed. Michel Foucault, the philosopher and social historian has been one of the most influential figures in this concept of 'social constructionism'. This rejects the assumption that, for example, mental illness is a fact or a 'reality' waiting to be discovered but that we construct the very meaning of certain behaviours by the way we talk and describe them, through the prevailing discourse. The differing accounts and definitions of health that were identified in the second chapter give an indication of the way that our understanding of health differs, depending on our experience and occupational role and that certain meanings predominate and begin to gain more influence.

The effect of labelling in any society serves to isolate difference or 'deviance' from the norm. Psychiatric labelling sets the ill person apart from the rest of us, the illness something we have or haven't got – a clear demarcation between mentally ill and mentally well, rather than seeing it as individual variation within broad boundaries of being a human being.

The women who formed the self-help group for mothers with depression expressed this in the following way:

'You're too scared to ask for help, so we cannae say what we want. We felt judged, felt blamed because we were not coping. It makes you feel awful.'

'It's really frightening to say what you feel. You think, if I tell her that, the bairns will get taken away. You're frightened of being labelled a bad mother. Mother and toddler groups are not the solution for these feelings.'

(Project Report)

In the field of mental health particularly, the process of defining health and ill health can be seen to be a much more complex process than at first sight. As workers in the field it is important to be critically aware of and understand our own perceptions and fears which we may be bringing as a sort of unconscious baggage which might direct the way we engage with people. The idea that some definitions might describe only one kind of reality, from a particular set of perspectives and that these are socially constructed and negotiated might free us to be more aware of the power relationships involved.

The Casualty Campaign

This second example moves away from the narrow concentration on individual relationships between doctors and patients and looks at the way the medical profession, or the 'professional monopolisers' as defined by Alford, operate to maintain and protect their powerful position and the effect this can have on service provision. This example uses the experience of the long campaign conducted by the Western General Action Group (WGAG), to retain a Casualty service in the local area.

One of the most persistent arguments for the closure of the casualty department in the local hospital rested on the definition of what this service was and who it was for and reflected the wider debates and conflicting views that were taking place on a national scale.

The changes of name for such services – from 'Casualty' to 'Accident and Emergency' to 'Minor Injuries Unit' reflect a struggle for the definition of emergency services which has been played out nationally since the late 1960's. Up until then, the casualty service was rather a neglected aspect of the National Health Service but in 1962 the Platt Report recommended that the service should be more centralised with Accident and Emergency Centres for more serious injuries attached to district general hospitals and smaller casualty departments serving peripheral areas. Emphasis was placed on the need to have skilled or 'specialist' hospital treatment to deal with serious injury and the proposed changes were seen by some as an attempt to impose the traditional model of hospital 'specialist' care onto the community emergency services. It has also been suggested that this change of policy reflected the influence of the orthopaedic surgeons who were concerned about creating centres where they could develop their specialist interests (Calnan 1982). In the event, this policy failed as people continued to use both A&E Centres and casualty departments for a wide variety of emergencies, some major and some minor.

Use of Emergency Services

In the years following this report, the use of A&E and casualty departments by the general public for a wide range of emergencies was increasingly seen as a problem by some doctors within the health service. Others felt that this was not a problem and that the casualty service should remain as a community medical emergency service available for a wider range of problems, rather than be developed into a separate specialist service only treating serious acute incidents.

'Patients in a social predicament cannot be turned away. Whatever form the "social predicament" may take – accommodating it must continue to be the raison d'être of a casualty service for the foreseeable future.'

(The Casualty Surgeons Association 1973)

Their view of what constitutes a community emergency service seems more in tune with the public's perception of an emergency, as we shall see later. However, the prestige and status of the casualty surgeons was overtaken during the 1980's and 1990's by the rise of A&E surgeons and the growth of major trauma as a new and highly specialised area of work. This changed the way emergency services were perceived, which was based on a view that a range of minor conditions and the need for support or reassurance or advice should be met by GP's or the primary health care team, not by a hospital service. This view continued to be put forward despite research which showed that most GP's were unable to provide such an emergency service and that many minor emergencies happened when people were not anywhere near their GP.

The new speciality of major trauma increased the ability to save severely injured people and dramatically improved the mortality rates for this group, particularly if patients could reach the specialised service as soon as possible. This led to the development of major trauma units, which contain a team of highly trained staff and sophisticated equipment. Television has perhaps encouraged the high profile and 'glamour' of white coated medics attending dramatic and severe accidents. The status and money involved in these units mean that resources have to be sucked in from other aspects of the service and the push to establish one of these major trauma centres in Edinburgh had a direct effect on the argument by the Health Board that the local Casualty Department at the Western General would have to close. It was this argument which led to the setting up of the local campaign.

These dilemmas are not new within the health service. Decisions have increasingly had to be taken to deal with the tension between developing expensive high tech services at the forefront of medicine and extending preventative services or treatment for chronic or disabling conditions which affect the majority of people. For example, of the 34,000 attendances at the local casualty department, only 1% required a high tech life saving facility. The Health Board's own research demonstrated the different needs presented by patients.

Severity of Injury	%	No
Requiring immediate, potentially life-saving intervention	1%	350
Other serious cases requiring admission	23%	8,000
Moderately severe (requiring X-ray)	43%	15,000
Minor cases not requiring X-ray	33%	11,000

CHAPTER 6

The Western General Action Group (WGAG) fully supported the need for seriously injured patients to have the treatment that was available in the centre of town but also wanted a service for the majority of local people – the bottom two groups in the above table – representing 76% of all attendances, 26,000 people, to be retained at the local hospital.

Some of these less serious cases would include people who need reassurance – parents who were scared by their child's condition and who might in the end only need advice or a kindly word. It would also include a small number of more vulnerable people, such as those who are homeless, or not able to register with a GP, who can often get the medical care they need at a Casualty Department. Traditionally, these departments have always provided this mix of medical, clinical, and informal social care as well as health advice and information.

'Inappropriate' Attenders and the Struggle for Definition

Research repeatedly shows that the majority of people use Casualty or A&E services because they can not get the help they need, at the time or the place where the incident occurred, anywhere else. Their own GP's do not have X-Ray facilities, or are unavailable after hours. Accidents can happen when people are miles away from home or their own doctor (Green, Dale 1992). The public, in other words, are defining casualty or accident and emergency services as those which they go to when something has happened which they define as serious and the circumstances in which it occurs mean that they cannot get help anywhere else. In this sense it is an emergency for them – a view supported by the old Casualty Surgeons Association, referred to earlier, who stated in 1973 that emergency situations were definable in terms of:

*'the **circumstances** in which incapacity from injury or illness occurs and do not imply that diagnosis is necessarily one requiring immediate intensive therapy.'*

Campaign leaflet.

WESTERN GENERAL ACTION GROUP
PROPOSED CLOSURE OF CHILDREN'S UNIT AND ACCIDENT AND EMERGENCY.
PUBLIC MEETING

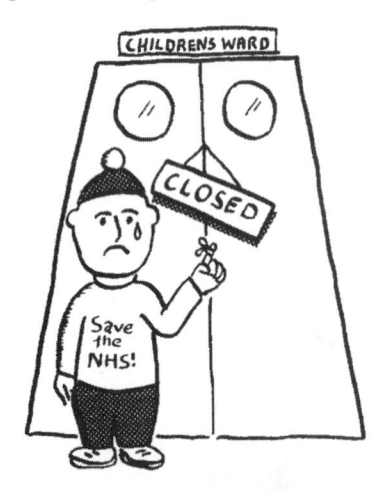

TUESDAY 24TH JANUARY
CRAIGROYSTON HIGH SCHOOL 7PM-9PM
CRECHE FACILITIES AVAILABLE

The health service on the other hand was beginning to re-define and restrict the use of casualty services as services for only those who are seriously or dangerously ill. Reports and articles in medical journals increasingly alluded to the problem of 'inappropriate attenders' who were seen to constitute a large group of attenders at A&E or Casualty Departments. Estimates of the size of this group varied between 30% and 40% of all attenders. These people were seen as not needing the specialist care that is available – they had 'minor' injuries and 'social problems' which should be dealt with elsewhere. Many of the debates and counter claims in relation to this issue represent a clash within the profession – of different medical interest groups. For example, a report written by a public health doctor in a city where local people occupied their local hospital's A&E department to prevent it being closed and centralised, stated:

'we would agree that the key to the problem is patients' perceptions but not that these perceptions are wrong and need changing. Most people given a choice between two services will choose the one that best meets their perceived needs. If the public are of the opinion that an A&E Dept. provides a treatment service for minor injuries that is more acceptable, accessible, equitable, effective, relevant and efficient than the only alternative, then we should not be surprised when they use it.'

(Garnett 1991)

The Lothian Health Board in the case of the Western General was therefore merely reflecting a dominant perspective in the 'resplendent hall of mirrors' within the health service which saw that only people requiring specialist medical attention or admission should come to an emergency service.

Professional Interests

Friedson's classic work on professions provides a basis for understanding the struggle for definition of this service (Friedson 1975). One of the key features which distinguishes a profession from other workers is the amount of autonomy granted to them to control their own sphere of work. Medicine in particular has achieved a high degree of professional autonomy. Within the profession, some groups are seen to have higher status than others and a significant aspect of this status and prestige is the extent to which a group can claim

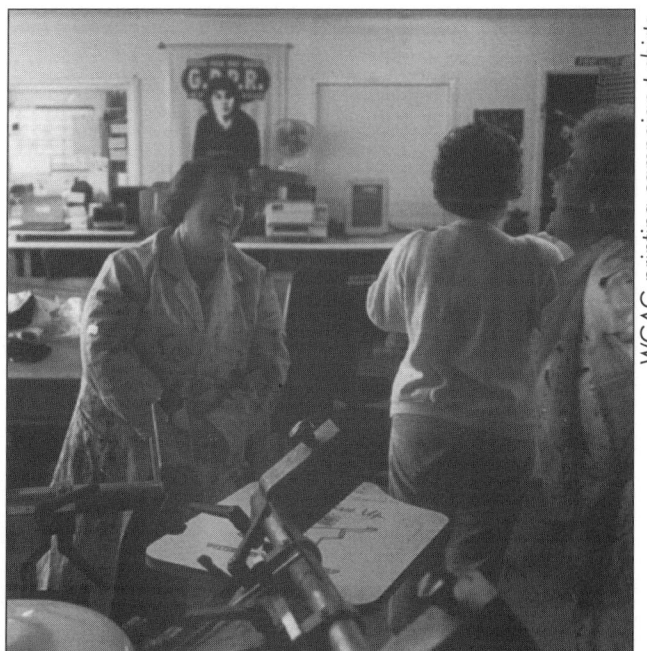

WGAG printing campaign t-shirts.

a specialist clinical area of work and control access to this.

The 'setting' of emergency services is at the interface of the hospital and the community. Unlike other medical specialities, which limit access through referral systems and appointments, patients can walk in off the street and expect treatment for a wide variety of injuries or complaints. The traditional use of casualty departments therefore limits the amount of control that doctors have over the patients that they see and consequently reduces their chance of specialising and achieving higher status within the profession. However the very nature of accidents, and the circumstances in which they occur, require this open accessibility.

Here we can see the roots of the tension behind different attempts to define 'emergency'. The definition of the function of an emergency service in turn defines 'appropriate' attendance. The power of some groups within the medical profession to define their own area of work has led them to define almost the majority of users of this service as inappropriate users.

'Because the helping professions define other people's status (and their own), the special terms they employ to categorise clients...... are especially revealing of the political functions language performs and of the multiple realities it helps to create.'

(Edelman 1974)

Although there are differences between groups of doctors, the polarity of views relating to emergency service can be summarised in the following diagram:

Patients View	Issues	Professional View
Perceived severity and context in which injury occurs	DEFINITION OF EMERGENCY	Severity of symptom
Wants open accessibility	ACCESS TO SERVICE	Control of access
Wide range of complaints and injuries	TYPE OF COMPLAINTS SEEN	Narrow, Specific, Serious injury
Free accessible and available service	CONCERNS	Specialism, expertise. Status linked to income
Complementary to	RELATIONSHIP TO GP SERVICE	Distinct and separate
Safety net if no other support available	USE OF CASUALTY FOR REASSURANCE	Inappropriate use Moral judgement

The meaning of what constituted an emergency service was being re-defined in order to establish a more specialist medical service which, while being justified in terms of the quality of care offered to patients with life-threatening injury, would also have the effect of extending hospital doctors' power and status. The WGAG were trying to ensure that the 'community interest' was articulated and put onto the official agenda where policy decisions were being taken. Before the WGAG began to form, the Health Board were heavily under the influence of the 'professional monopolisers', the medics. They were exercising their power through their 'expert knowledge', their status and authority, and by the influence they had by the positions they held – both on the Board, in attendance at Board meetings, by influencing the executive officers and through the area medical committees. All these positions they hold within the decision making structures are a symbol of the power they enjoy which is, in the main, supported by society.

The Effects on people

Two years into the campaign, the Health Board eventually decided to close the local Casualty Department. Emergency services for the people of Edinburgh were to be provided for people with relatively serious injuries or illness from one A&E Department in the centre of town. It would be located in the same department as the major trauma unit so that if this highly specialised help was required it would be instantly available. This meant that when a serious case was admitted, people with less severe injuries such as a broken arm or bad cut would have to wait while the department concentrated on the more serious case – the triage system. The waiting times at this central unit increased to 5, 6 and 7 hours, in a significant minority of cases. When the local casualty department had closed, the majority of people who had used it, approximately 23,000 people per year, had to join the queues of people from the rest of the city at this one central department. Staff in this central department expressed their concern privately to the WGAG that they just could not cope.

The WGAG were inundated with stories of bad treatment and long waiting times which were compiled into a dossier entitled 'Casualties of Indifference'. The WGAG summarised the effects on local people: 'Along with patients from the rest of the city, the people of north Edinburgh now have a worse service because they:

- **have to travel further and wait longer**
- **are experiencing a worse service at the overstretched Sick Kids and Royal Infirmary hospitals.**
- **are not getting basic injuries such as fractures properly identified and treated.**
- **are as a consequence, suffering pain for a lot longer than is acceptable.**
- **are having to pay more in travel costs.'**

The tenacity of the WGAG in continuing to lobby members of the Health Board, in submitting reports of the effects of the centralised service, produced unease amongst

CHAPTER 6

some members of the Board and gradually amongst many health professionals. This began to swing support away from the previously dominant group.

A New Alliance of Interests

The clash over the definition of the service enabled the WGAG to understand some of the influences on the way services are planned and delivered. They accordingly lobbied both individual doctors and consultants and the profession's influential area medical committees and tried to make their power more visible and the conflict of interests more public. They began to meet with individual members of the Board to force a split in the apparent consensus. They also managed, at times, to persuade other groups of medics such as the GP's and individual hospital doctors, to support the community interest and they built up massive local support in the community and in the local press. They worked to attract cross party support. especially in the run up to the General Election, received support from the regional and district councils and wrote to Health Ministers at the Scottish Office.

This activity delayed the decision to close the local casualty department for over two years until finally, the Health Board slipped their decision through during a Trades holiday, at a venue out of town, when a number of supporters, including Board members, of the 'community interest' happened to be on holiday or absent. The local health council only received the agenda of this meeting the evening before – after they had closed their offices at the end of the day.

The campaign continued and the Health Board tried to pacify this protest by providing a small scale service for a few hours a day in a local clinic, much against the wishes of local people. This was very poorly used and there were increasing workload problems in the A&E department in the centre of town.

The WGAG travelled to other parts of the country, looking at other alternative models of emergency care and at the end of the campaign were instrumental in identifying a Minor Injury Service based in London which was run by nurse practitioners. The advantages to the group were clear. The unit provided an X-ray and plastering service, was open 12 hours a day, 7 days a week and had clear guidelines about how to deal with more serious conditions. It was felt that this would clearly satisfy the needs of the community in north west Edinburgh.

During the campaign, the Western General Hospital moved to trust status and its management structure changed accordingly. The new management was particularly interested in the London model of a minor injuries unit. It represented a cheaper and more effective service for minor injuries than the old casualty model with highly paid doctors on call. The Trust also wanted an emergency service in the hospital so that it could attract patients and bring in income. This more managerial, market perspective can be seen as representing the 'corporate rationalisers' who wanted above all, value for money!

Another professional group, the nurses within the hospital, also supported this move as it offered more specialist training for themselves and so satisfied their own particular professional interests.

The north west area of Edinburgh covered two political constituencies, a safe Labour seat and a marginal Tory held seat. The Labour MP Malcolm Chisholm had always actively supported the WGAG and during the last year of the campaign organised a deputation from the campaign to meet with the Scottish Office Minister for Health. The campaign became a key issue for the marginal constituency and it received support from all candidates. The declining support for the Tories in Scotland at that time meant that the campaign became a crucial issue in the run up to the General Election in 1992. Michael Forsyth who was then Minister for Health, instructed the NHS Executive in Scotland to encourage Lothian Health Board to review their decision to close the Casualty Department at the Western General Hospital.

This new alliance of different interest groups – the 'corporate rationalisers' in the Trust, the nurses in the hospital and the politicians, combined to challenge the dominant medical professional view and enabled the campaign to push the Health Board to provide this local service once again at the Western General Hospital.

The learning from this experience was how little power the 'community interest' has in its own right. Hardly any of the professional interest groups described above seemed to have the interests of the community as their main priority

except for a small number of individuals, such as the local GP who had the courage to speak out strongly at a public meeting, and a public health doctor who provided the campaign with research data. A few of the lay members of the Health Board were also unhappy with the way the decision was being made and supported the WGAG's case, but were often in the minority and therefore usually out-voted at Board meetings. Local councillors had relatively little influence over the Health Board's decisions.

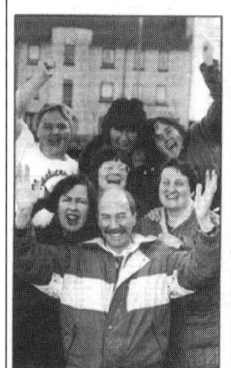

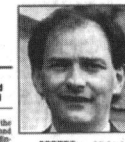

The members of the campaign were often incensed by the injustice that allowed a handful of people, representatives of the medical profession and some of the Board members, who were unelected and unaccountable to decide on an issue that affected so many people. In representing the 'community interest', the campaign was always well supported by local people, despite the Board at first trying to imply they were just a bunch of trouble makers, as can be seen by the extract below.

The campaign played a crucial role in keeping the issue alive and in the public eye by a constant barrage of creative and publicly supported demonstrations, community picnics, and other publicity stunts and building a huge array of community support. Its own power was through promoting this community view, marshalling a rational and moral argument and then persuading, lobbying, and shaming these more powerful groups to build a service around people's needs. However this form of power was quite ephemeral and at the end of the day, dependent on forming alliances with other powerful groups. They gradually managed to affect the decision making process opportunistically by spotting moments when interests converged and creating temporary alliances. Once the decision was made to re-instate a minor injuries service at the Western, the group were seen to have some power and were asked by the hospital management to become involved with creating links between the hospital and the local

---

A case for Casualty, 1993.

THE WESTERN GENERAL ACTION GROUP

The WGAG sincerely represents the views of the vast majority of users of the health services in north west Edinburgh. In this role the WGAG represents those for whom the service is supposed to be provided for – patients, users and consumers. The Patients' Charter and NHS White Paper both support the right of people as patients to have their views taken seriously.

With regard to the withdrawal of A&E services at the Western the WGAG has the support of:

- **over 12,000 people who signed petitions to retain the service**
- **letters from 21 local schools**
- **letters of support from local GP's and health visitors**
- **local clergy who serve the communities of Drylaw, Muirhouse, West Pilton and West Granton**
- **The Edinburgh Presbytery of the Church of Scotland**
- **MP's from all four major parties**

- **Regional councillors from all major parties**
- **Lothian Health Service Trade Union Committee**
- **Local industry such as GEC Ferranti**
- **Local branches of Scottish Old Age Pensioners Association (SOAPA)**
- **Local meetings and fund-raising events have regularly attracted 2-300 people**
- **Local mother and toddler groups from Davidsons Mains to Muirhouse, community groups, local shop keepers**
- **Staff from within the Western General Hospital**

community. This honeymoon period was brief. A year later, when the hospital celebrated the success of 'their' minor injuries unit in a public relations exercise, there was no mention of how it had been won by the efforts of the WGAG for the local community.

Conclusion

These two examples show some of the elements in the dynamics of power and how it affects people's lives. Power becomes entrenched in social relations through a complex process. We individually support the power of doctors to decide if we are ill, out of a need for 'expert' knowledge which can reduce our fear and uncertainty when we are sick and vulnerable, and for legitimation of this 'sick role'. Collectively we support this regulatory role in order that society can function smoothly. We are part of creating and responding to structures which respond to our needs as individuals and as a society.

The way in which these powerful roles are themselves regulated or made accountable determines whether the role is extended into other areas of our lives and how much individuals are constrained by them.

In the absence of a democratically accountable health service, the WGAG campaign can be seen as an attempt by individuals to try and challenge and change the structural and cultural support for medical dominance which allows the medical profession to extend their jurisdiction over the planning and provision of health services. Their interests became more visible, once the WGAG began to articulate the 'community voice'. The failure of this dominant group to keep the item off the official agenda meant they had to resort to other tactics in order to keep control. The presence of the community campaign meant that these twists and turns were noted and monitored and in this way made more public.

The eventual success of the campaign was important for the WGAG and the community. It demonstrated that power did not always remain with 'the Big Yins'. The skills, knowledge and experience gained at an individual level increased people's self-confidence and belief in their ability to influence events in their lives. The group's skills in developing strategies, building a community organisation and understanding how power is exercised has been utilised in other campaigns to promote the 'community interest' in health. The importance of the learning process alongside these experiences is examined in the next chapter.

References

Adams, L and Pintus, S (1994)	A challenge to prevailing theory and practice, Critical Public Health Vol.5:2, pp 17-28
Alford, Robert R (1975)	Health Care Politics, Ideological and Interest Group Barriers to Reform. University of Chicago Press
Calman, M (1982)	The Hospital Accident and Emergency Department: What is its Role?, Journal of Social Policy, 11, pp 483-502
Casualty Surgeons Association (1973)	An Integrated Emergency Service
Farrant, W (1991)	Health Promotion and Community Health Action in the UK, International Journal of Health Services, 21(3), pp 423-439
Freidson, E (1975)	The Profession of medicine: A study of the sociology of Applied Knowledge. Dodd Mead, New York
Foucault (1980)	Power and Knowledge, ed, Gordon, C. Harvester Press, Brighton
Garnet, Dr S (1992)	A Treatment Service for Minor Injuries: maintaining Equity of Access. North Manchester Health Authority
Green, J and Dale, J (1992)	Primary Care in Accident and Emergency and General Practice, Soc. Sci. Med., Vol.35 No.8, pp 987-995
Horwitz, A (1983)	The Social Control of Mental Illness. Academic Press, New York
Goffman, E (1961)	Asylums. Penguin, Harmondsworth
Goffman, E (1963)	Stigma: Notes on the Management of Spoiled Identity. Spectrum Books, Englewood Cliffs, New Jersey
Kobasa, S, Maddi, S and Kahn, S (1982)	Hardiness and Health: A Prospective Study, Journal of Personality and Social Psychology, Vol.42. No.1, pp 168-177
Lukes, S (1974)	Power: A radical view. Macmillan, London

McCormack, C (1993)	From the Fourth World to the Third World – A Common Vision of Health, Community Development Journal, Vol 28 No.3. OUP
Navarro, V (1984)	A critique of the ideological and political position of the Willy Brandt report and the WHO Alma Ata Declaration, Social Science and medicine, Vol.18 No.6, pp 467-474
Parsons, T (1951)	The Social System. Free Press of Glencoe, New York
Research Unit for Health and Behavioural Change (RUHBC) (1989)	Changing the Public Health, pp 43-4. John Wiley and Sons, Edinburgh University
Rotter, J B (1966)	Generalised expectancies for internal versus external control reinforcement, Psychological Monographs, 80 (1)
Rowbotham, S (1973)	Woman's Consciousness, Man's World. Pelican
Scheff, T (1966)	Being Mentally Ill: A Sociological Theory. Aldine Publishing Co, Chicago
Stainton Rogers, W (1993)	From Psychometric Scales to Cultural Perspectives. Open University and Macmillan
Wallerstein, N (1992)	Powerlessness, Empowerment, and Health: Implications for Health Promotion Programmes, American Journal of Health Promotion, Vol.6 No.3, Jan/Feb 1992
Williamson, C (1988)	Dominant, Challenging and Repressed Interests in the NHS, Health Services Management, December 1988
Wright Mills, C (1968)	The Sociological Imagination. Oxford University Press

Pilton Health Project Reports

After You Leave the Surgery	Video available from Pilton Video Project
Behind the Painted Smile	Report from the SHAME Group
A Case For Casualty	Report by the WGAG

We Make the Road by Walking

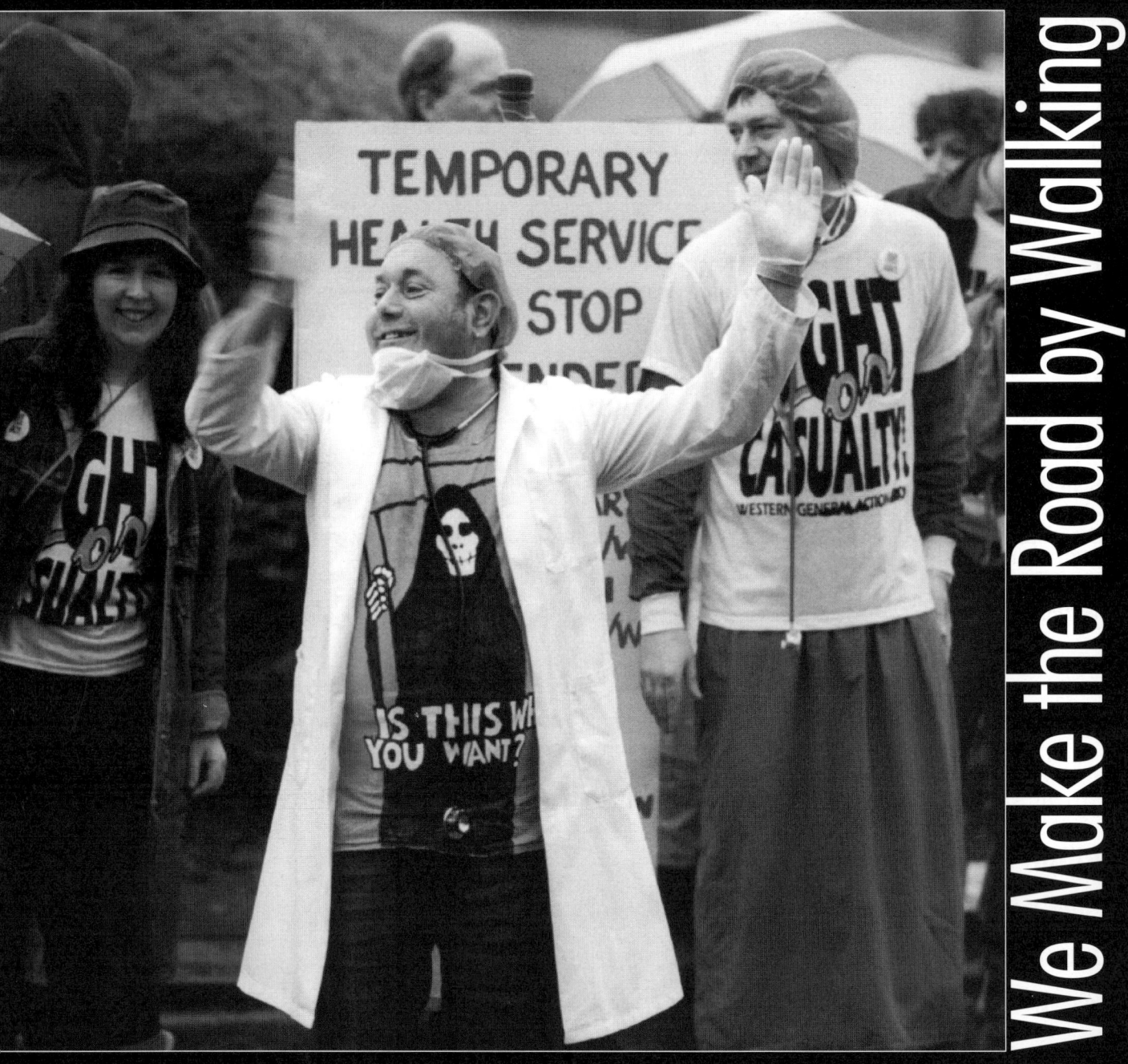

Conducting the traffic at the Casualty Closure Demonstration, Western General Hospital

Introduction

In the initial stages of the project, when we were meeting local people for the first time, we described the Pilton project as a community health project, not as a health education project. We were aware of people's feelings about some of the more traditional health education approaches which were perceived as telling people to adopt healthier lifestyles while taking no account of the context of their lives. The 'victim blaming' aspect to a number of national publicity campaigns at that time in the early 1980's also served to give people in working class areas a sceptical and negative view of education in relation to health and although we were very aware of the educational role within community development, we wished to distance ourselves from this more negative image and to meet people on our own terms.

The form of health education which we were unwilling to be associated with was that which imposed a particular, dominant view onto people. Paulo Freire, the Brazilian adult educator and philosopher called this the 'banking' method of education, in which the teacher is seen as possessing all the knowledge and information and transmits this to students or pupils. Pupils are seen as passive and as 'empty vessels' waiting to be filled with this knowledge. Freire's view of education is that it is about liberation, not domestication and that the process is about working with people to become more critical, creative, free and active members of society. In this sense it is seen as an essential part of social change and transformation.

Many of the different activities we became engaged with, included developing learning programmes with group members, both formally and informally. An evaluation of the Health Project in 1992 remarked on the way that local residents involved with the project valued the educative aspect of the work. In a workshop facilitated by the evaluator, participants were asked to respond to the question – what for you are the most important things this project is trying to achieve? The report noted that the item on 'improving knowledge' prompted much discussion. In particular, it was local residents who insisted on its importance. They emphasised that they valued 'learning from each other on their own terms, in an informal way and also from outside invited experts' (Beattie 1992).

The ideas and philosophy of Freire were an enormous source of inspiration and encouragement as we developed our own practice (Freire 1985). We were fortunate in being able to learn more about his ideas and to examine the implications for practice through the Adult Learning Project (ALP) in Edinburgh. Since 1979, the ALP project has been developing and adapting Freirian methods within an urban Scottish context and have been willing to share their progress and thinking with other practitioners in a variety of ways. Initially there were a number of discussions with the

ALP workers, Stan Reeves and Gerri Kirkwood about this approach and once Christa, the health visitor joined the project we both attended their practitioner exchange meetings regularly over a number of years. These meetings enabled us to share our thinking and explore how we could put this into practice and the ALP project remained an important intellectual and practical resource.

The bigger story of the development of ALP has now been written (Kirkwood, G & Kirkwood C, 1989). Freire's ideas about education and the humanisation of society has also been influential for many years in the health programmes of developing countries (Hope, A, Timmel, S and Hodzi, C. 1986), (Macdonald, J. 1993), and more recently in the West, as a practical method of tackling powerlessness and inequity in health (Wallerstein, N 1993).

Earlier chapters have explored the development of our own thinking as we listened to local people talk about their own lives and concerns – the importance of the relationship, the act of listening, the struggle for definition and meaning, and the impact of power and control on genuine dialogue. The ideas of Freire found a resonance with this experience of listening for 'themes' or those issues which people felt strongly about.

This chapter takes a number of key ideas which heavily influenced our thinking and together with case studies attempts to demonstrate how we translated these into our own practice.

Dialogue

Freire uses this term in the sense of real communication between people. Kirkwood describes it as the communication that occurs between people who are genuinely thinking and working together on some aspect of their lived reality (1989). It implies a reciprocal process in which individuals can feel free to share, listen to and learn from, each others' experience. No one has all the answers and no one is totally ignorant – it is a mutual learning process.

The essence of these ideas permeated the health project activities. For example, in our attempt to encourage active participation in the planning and delivery of services, we were interested in creating opportunities for a more genuine dialogue between people so that they could begin to work out what they wanted from the service providers, rather than just reacting to someone else's agenda. Too often, a tokenistic form of 'consultation with the community' takes place which does not draw on lay people's knowledge in an effective way. One off public meetings, organised in a traditional format with the 'experts' on a platform, literally 'talking down to' the assembled large audience, does not encourage a meaningful exchange. Similarly, individual questionnaires or surveys which contain only questions which are considered important by service providers, can only scratch the surface of the wealth of knowledge and information which could be utilised. Encouraging genuine dialogue and participation takes more time and requires relationships built on trust and respect.

The problematic nature of community participation has been clearly described by Sherry Arnstein who uses the analogy of a 'ladder' of citizen participation. She suggests that most activities undertaken under the banner of participation are meaningless and only the top three 'rungs' involve genuine attempts at citizen power. The concept of 'dialogue' in the Freirian sense supports a move up the ladder towards partnership, rather than the rather limited process of public consultation.

The Ladder of Participation

Citizen Control
Delegated Power   Degrees of citizen power
Partnership
Placation
Consultation   Degrees of Tokenism
Informing
Therapy   Non-participation
Manipulation

(Arnstein, 1969)

Example: The Tranquillisers Group seeking Information

As part of planning the group programme, members of the Tranquillisers Support Group 'Come Off It!' wanted to know more about the effect of tranquillisers on their bodies and aspects of their treatment in psychiatric hospital. Two of the questions they wanted answered were, what tranquillisers do in your body and why did they have to attend patient reviews when they were in hospital?

This search for information can be seen as part of the action/reflection cycle – at the point when people are encouraged to ask – What do we know? What do we need to know? – and to invite outside experts to share their knowledge. The challenge of organising this type of interaction is to create a truly dialogical experience with people mutually exploring a subject as equal experts.

A psychiatrist who was not working in the local sector, was invited to come to the group and help us with these questions from his professional perspective. The worker's role in this situation was to create a type of 'level playing field' so that the imbalance of power was reduced as much as possible and the group could benefit from the knowledge of the professional expert and draw him into their own exploration of the issue. The meeting took place in the local community centre where the group met – where they were comfortable in their own territory. A pre-meeting established and clarified the key questions the group wanted asked, and the questions were written up on a large piece of flipchart paper as a reminder and to keep the group to task. Those who offered to ask the main questions were then more confident in putting forward the queries that the whole group had identified although this did not preclude others joining in. This was important to establish as people were anxious about talking in this way to someone from a profession that they had all had very mixed experiences of. In this way, the opportunity for a more genuine dialogue was created. The psychiatrist answered the 'but why?' questions clearly and fairly.

CHAPTER 7

Firstly, he explained how tranquillisers worked to damp down the brain's normal activity. A number of people in the group were genuinely astonished by this information. They had thought that the drugs worked to somehow make them feel better, not to stop their brain working in certain ways. They also felt, in later discussions, that if they had known this at the time they had been prescribed medication, they might have decided not to take them at all. Some people were not informed that they were even being prescribed tranquillisers.

'I don't remember anything about tranquillisers. I actually thought the wee blue tablets were vitamin tablets until I saw the programme on TV.'

(Project Report, 1986)

The next question was about patient 'reviews' in psychiatric hospital. People's experience of these were that they were invited into a room with a lot of other people who they did not always know and were not always introduced to. They thought these people must all be doctors. Their case was then discussed by this large group of people as though they were not there and sometimes they felt completely disregarded in the ensuing discussion. They felt anxious and humiliated by this process. Their questions were 'What was the purpose of these? Who were all the people who attended? Who were they for?'

The psychiatrist explained that attendance at patients reviews was not just by doctors but other professional staff such as social workers, psychologists, and psychiatric nurses. The group then asked why all these people who did not know them were there and as he began to spell out the reasons for this it was apparent that reviews were primarily a means of training for the psychiatric team. The members of the group felt that this seemed to be the main purpose and expressed their view that for them it had little value and indeed was a source of anxiety. A useful review for them would be conducted in a very different manner. Both parties listened to each other thoughtfully.

Observing this dialogue, it was apparent that group members had not had the chance to ask this question so clearly before and it seemed as though the psychiatrist had not therefore been prompted to think about it from the patient's perspective before. The idea or meaning of what reviews were had grown out of the training needs of the profession, and were not usually questioned. Certain assumptions had been made about the usefulness of them for patients. It can, of course be argued, that this process ultimately benefits patients but maybe this connection has become rather tenuous because there has been little attempt to check this assumption with those for whom the service is for.

The learning opportunity for group members to untangle their own feelings and understandings from 'official accounts' was a key element in the group's development and self-confidence. Self-help groups can offer members a great deal of support but in community development practice it is also important to create opportunities for learning and for a critical examination of personal experiences in relation to broader social forces. Otherwise,

'mere expression of solidarity among people in similar states of powerlessness may lead to drowning in common despair'.

(Rees, 1991)

Naming the World

In the process of engaging in dialogue, sharing ideas and developing new meanings, words are crucial. They are an important part of the way we interact with our world – our private or public account – and the link this has with relationships and power. Our use of language, then, is extremely complex and varies in different situations. The use of the Scots and English language in Scotland is an obvious example of the way that power relations determine the language used. Hearing and using people's own words was an important part of the learning, for both local people and workers, as we explored issues together. The experience of seeing their exact words written up on a large flipchart, or in discussion notes, was a very powerful experience for some people, particularly if their views had not often been listened to or valued before. For the whole group it added a richness and an authenticity as well as a sense of ownership of the learning process. Freire saw the importance of 'naming the world' as you have experienced it, in your own terms and in your own language as an essential part of shaping it. This concept, which at first seemed fairly straightforward, seemed to grow in importance and complexity as we began to see how it connected with different aspects of our work.

Three of these are presented here:–
- **Defining your own reality**
- **The use of language**
- **Creative expression**

Defining Your Own Reality

As we have discussed earlier, the use of definitions or labels can be seen as an instrument of social control whereby the dominant way of describing the world is imposed on others. The act of naming the world as you experience it, in your own terms, is a process of acting on the world, not just accepting it as it is. Freire describes the way that people who he describes as the oppressed – the dispossessed, the colonised or the marginalised – are treated as 'objects' in a way which denies their humanity. He believes people should be seen as 'subjects' who can know and engage with the world about them.

Freire believed that naming the world is everyone's right, not the privilege of the few. He felt that you needed to name the world in dialogue with others and that this was not just about words alone but was about developing a more critical analysis, involving reflection and action, of your own experience in the wider world.

The following example shows how one group, by sharing their own reality of depression associated with childbirth, began to re-define the meaning of this for themselves.

Example: Work on 'Post-natal Depression'

A support group for women who had been identified as suffering from post-natal depression was established by the project health visitor in collaboration with a colleague. Gradually, two local women who had been group members began to take over the running of the group. Initially the health visitors had called the group the 'Post-natal Support Group' but the women felt unhappy with this name and decided to change the name to 'Self Help Around Mum's Experiences' (S.H.A.M.E.). The project worker's role here was to explore the reasons behind this rather than be defensive about a change of name and to encourage the women to express and reflect on their feelings about the labelling of post-natal depression and this was a thread which ran through group meetings alongside their other task of supporting each other. The importance of their analysis was again supported and encouraged by holding a structured discussion of their experience of depression which was recorded, written up so that they could add comments or criticisms and finally produced as a report, 'Behind a Painted Smile'. (S.H.A.M.E., 1991). The report is a powerful critique of how post-natal depression is usually understood. It challenges the way it is defined and dealt with within the health service.

The first stage in this process of re-definition was the decision by the women to change the name of the group – because by this time it was **their** group. They were running it and they felt more in control. The process of listening and sharing experiences with other women had legitimised their belief that the 'official' definition of this experience represented a very partial view.

The selection of words in the new name that was adopted conveys a shift in who is in control of the definition. From a diagnostic label – 'post-natal depression', coined by experts, to a name for the group which firmly places it within their control – in 'self help', based on their own knowledge, and trusting their own experience – 'mums' experience'.

Their re-definition of post-natal depression developed over some months as their shared views were discussed, refined and sounded out in the group. Some of the more traditional medical explanations – about a change in hormone levels were seen as being too narrow. The label which signifies **when** the depression occurs, that is post-natal, after the birth, was also challenged as being too simplistic and they broadened this to include an understanding of the total significance of becoming a parent. The whole context within which becoming pregnant and having a child takes place was brought into their analysis, including the symbolic meaning attached to new life and its connection with death.

The question that they first addressed was – what is post-natal depression? The group identified four contributing factors: the loss of identity; not coping anymore; coping with loss or bereavement; and a life crisis.

The Loss of Identity

'First of all we have doubts about whether we exist at all after giving birth! As soon as you open your door and you're going out with your pram, your next door neighbour comes out and says "what a lovely baby!" The downstairs neighbour comes out and its "Hello beautiful, and how are you this morning? Did she sleep all night?" Then the next one "Oh look at her wee shoes" and the next one "Oh she's coming on". You get home and sit there waiting for your partner and he comes in and says "Where's the bairn? Is she sleeping? Has she been fed? Does she need changed?" – all in one breath and on and on it goes.

Is this post-natal depression – that the woman, that mum becomes invisible?'

Not Coping Anymore

More importantly we think it's something to do with giving and loving, sharing and caring until you cannot, anymore. You suffer when you cannot give anymore. For some of us this is also linked to our own lack of mothering when we were children. Behind that painted smile, mum is not getting any tender loving care.

'There are so many faces we put on. The knots in the stomach are so tight but you daren't say you can't cope.'

Coping with Loss

In our group we have discovered that as well as a lack of mothering, there have been other losses too. The loss can have been the death of a previous baby, a miscarriage, a termination, a boyfriend. Whatever it may have been, it is equally important to the individual and the pain is unbearable. The pain becomes worse when you have a new baby to cope with, whether it happened last year or ten years ago.

'As a 16 year old my home was a very ordinary one, with both parents and a brother living with me. An older brother, wife and niece, visiting lots. My house was never empty. My mother was then diagnosed as having cancer. It took 2 years waiting, just waiting on her dying. These were silent years, very, very quiet years. In February my mother died. In August my father left for Arizona. I fell pregnant and the baby's father left. My baby was born, his father came back then left again very quickly. I had met my health visitor during pregnancy who was very kind, supportive and everything I wanted. However, she wasn't there when Gavin was born. Gavin died 7 weeks later. My health visitor was on holiday. I had to go it alone. I buried that little darling of mine – dealing with everything you have to as head of a family. (What family I find myself saying). My two brothers lived together and I lived on in the ghost house which seemed like a shadow of the one I used to know. I didn't want to go to Arizona. I didn't want to terminate my baby. I didn't want him to die. Nor my mum – but I did make my bed. I knew I had to lie in it.

I went on to marry Gavin's father. I was high as a kite. Happiness at last I thought – my nightmare was over. I was so desperate for another baby. However, during my pregnancy I cried myself to sleep, hysterically every night for no reason. Steadily things got worse. I gave birth to a 9lb baby boy – the picture of health. My nightmare was just beginning. To say the least, on his first birthday and when he took his first steps, I was a patient in the Royal Edinburgh Hospital.'

A Life Crisis

Having a baby certainly is a huge change – in our situation and in our feelings.

'Your whole life changes. I never thought you'd be that extreme, but you are. You have these feelings. Sometimes it can be "I hate you" about the baby but you're frightened to say it.'

'Once you've had the baby, the professionals think that's OK – but some women do hate their baby for a time. You're feeling like shit and the last thing you want to do is look after a baby.'

'Sometimes you just want to throw the toys out of the window with the kids attached.'

'I can remember trying to tell my family about post-natal depression and they said "you've got to love it and get on with your life". I don't know if they were frightened or what but I couldn't talk to them about it.'

The report then went on to examine some of the assumptions around post-natal depression and motherhood. That having a baby means you are an adult. That if you have other children, you'll have no problems. That post-natal depression begins after birth.

'I started taking post-natal depression much later – about 6-7 months later.'

'It began before I had my baby. It doesn't just happen after birth.'

Naming these experiences and critically reflecting on their collective meaning produced a different reality to the dominant view or meaning given to post-natal depression. The fact that this perspective is not on the official agenda has serious implications for the way services are organised and how much they can help women who experience depression related to having a baby.

Firstly, the services are not available if a woman's 'post-natal' depression starts too early or too late! Because the official definition filters through into the public's understanding, other support and help from social networks might also not be easily utilised. In other words, a friend or family member might 'recognise' depression after childbirth and offer support or seek help but if it happens at the wrong time it might go unnoticed. The woman herself, of course, internalises these official definitions and if her experience doesn't fit – she can feel even more distressed and alone. Secondly, if some of the feelings around this event are not understood, measures of help and support, which might be relatively simple to offer or provide are not brought into play and more serious distress could develop which could have been prevented.

A video made by members of the Middle House Stress Centre also touched on this sense of disjuncture between their own and health professionals definitions or diagnoses and the effect this had on honest communication.

'I visualise them as having to look up those wee text books and if it wasnae in there it didn't exist! They didn't treat you on a one to one basis, as a person – I think they used their own thoughts and the way they think about things as that's how things must be.'

'They've got to have a pattern and to show that this pattern's working – whether it's working or not and sometimes you say to the doctor – aye, you're feeling well, when you're not really – just to get it over with. It's not a truthful thing, because you learn you know – you get to learn what they want to hear and you give them it.'

(After you leave the Surgery, 1989)

The Use of Language

The dramatic changes in British society, initiated by the Thatcher government created a new language and a new discourse. Throughout the late 1980's and 1990's market economics and the rise of the entrepreneurial approach to public services created a bizarre language of business terms juxtaposed onto words with the 'feel good' factor such as 'care packages' and 'quality controllers'. The appointment pages of health journals became awash with adverts looking for business development/marketing managers, costing assistants, and financial controllers to work within the health service.

As new words appeared, others disappeared. For a while, 'poverty' did not exist anymore and it disappeared in official health documents. The 'Health of the Nation' document produced in 1992, referred to 'variations' in health amongst socio-economic groups rather than 'inequalities' at a time when research revealed that the widening of inequalities in health since 1979 mirrored the gross upwards redistribution of wealth that had occurred in the UK (British Medical Journal editorial 1994).

Linguistic theory has long supported the view that language, thought and action shape each other.

'Language is always an intrinsic part of some particular social situation; it is never an independent instrument or simply a tool for description. By naively perceiving it as a tool, we mask its profound part in creating social relationships and in evoking the roles and the "selves" of those involved in the relationships.'

(Edelman 1974)

Foucault, among others has suggested that the essence of power is to participate in, influence or even take control of the dominant discourse. This can also involve contesting the language by which power is expressed (Rees 1991). The following is an example of how we tried to tackle the numbing effect of the use of this new language in relation to the NHS Reforms.

Changes in the NHS – Listening to Local Voices

Contesting the language and insisting on entering into this discourse, was the purpose of the 'Listening to Local Voices' Conference which looked at changes in the NHS. All of us, workers and local residents felt dis-empowered by the jargon describing the changes in the health service that began to take place in 1991.

'part of the problem was that the complexities of the new arrangements and the jargon that was being used, served to make people feel stupid and therefore unwilling to engage with the issue. A first step was to admit that we all felt like this – workers and committee and local people! The new health-speak of "provider/purchaser splits", "trusts", and "internal markets" felt like a foreign language and we were conscious of how powerful some people felt in speaking in this new way – even if they didn't fully understand it themselves!'

(Who is Listening to Local Voices, 1993)

Weeks before the conference, a number of informal workshops were organised, with the prime aim of de-mystifying the jargon surrounding the changes and using straightforward language and role play to describe what seemed to be happening. As part of the evaluation of the whole conference we asked people what they had felt about attending these informal workshops before-hand.

'It gave me a better idea of the changes that Trusts and opting out really means'

'I found the workshops very helpful as I had little knowledge of what the changes would mean'.

'I understood a bit more what was happening and it helped me to join in more'.

Presenters, facilitators and panel members were all instructed to speak in clear direct language, to avoid or explain jargon or short hand terms. Participants were also urged to speak up if they did not understand any of the new terms – and they did. Managers were questioned about the lack of accountability of the trusts, the composition of trust boards, the pressure for pay beds and national pay agreements. Other groups discussed the issues of the reforms on more vulnerable groups, such as the elderly and those with a disability. A debate in the afternoon raised the question of rights, and whether 'expensive' patients would be struck off a doctor's list. The conference also expressed a concern that money would become the prime consideration in the NHS and that this would affect relationships between people and the medical profession. Once the meaning of this particular language had been explored and sometimes challenged and there was a basic understanding of what the reforms meant, people engaged in an energetic debate and began to critically assess the implications for themselves.

Creative Expression

Various forms of creative expression can sometimes uncover a way to name both our individual or unique experience as well as our collective and common ones. It can often help to unlock us from a form of language which can be seen as belonging to the dominant group. Creative writing, poetry, songs, sketches and making videos and slide/tape presentations were part of this process.

Poems from the Middle House Stress Centre

Ageing

God preserve me from sheepskin coats and fur coats,
and from blue rinses and becoming an old goat,
From all my fears of loneliness,
The regrets and grey hairs, and the terror of illness,
loss of mind and steep stairs

Oh let me tell the truth about my age
If anyone asks, that is,
And accept that my children are adults,
Though to me they're my kids.

I don't care what you think, I still feel young inside
I've had so much experience, why should I hide?
I will not conform to your image of me,
I shall grow old gracefully, feeling content and free.

Elsie, Margaret, Wilma, Anne and Catherine

Middle House

Middle House between Ainslie Park
and Ferranti

Wee cup o' tea, better than your Auntie,
Discussion groups and meetings
Caring and also sharing
Walks and talks, relaxes stress
We'll help you get out of a mess

Relaxation and taping
To ease body, mind and spirit from aching
Communal dinner and tea
You're left to yourself
to be.

Walter

CHAPTER 7

Making Slide/Tape Presentations

When the women's health discussion group decided to look at the issue of damp housing and health in more depth they made a slide/tape presentation. This involved taking photos, and making transparencies out of them which are then projected onto a screen, accompanied by a taped sound commentary – the kind of thing seen in museums or historic houses. This was seen as a means of getting their ideas across to a wider audience but it also involved them in a creative and educational process. Constructing a slide/tape programme meant the group had to spend a lot of time planning what they wanted to say, constructing a logical progression of ideas, prioritising different aspects and finding out more information. This then had to be taped and edited. Photos had to be decided on, taken and developed and both these and the sound tape assembled into a coherent whole. Group members interviewed the local housing manager, the local GP, a councillor and a union representative. Community Education provided funding for a slide/tape tutor, Pete Gregson to come and work with us.

The whole process involved a great deal of discussion and decision making and the authenticity of the end programme had an immediate impact on those who watched it (Home Sweet Home, 1985). At the beginning of the following year, the group were invited to show the video as part of a seminar programme at Edinburgh University which led to the research into the effects of damp

---

Poems from the Tranquillisers Group

Making Changes

Here's my recipe
My ensurance for success

Pick up the pieces
Not to worry
If you don't have all the ingredients
Find a friend
To stir the pot

Step by Step, get yourself out
Mix with others
Stir slowly now, don't be afraid
Rise a little at a time
Take care to remember ...
... your special mixture
Add a bit more to the crowd
Taste, you might like it.
Sprinkle some spice with your friend
Take turns to blend
Bring to a slow simmer
Now and again, peek in the oven door
To check the progress
If you think you've succeeded
You can do it some more

Arlene

Pills, Pills, Pills

Morning and night
Blue, yellow, red, brown and white
Little devils they are
How did it start?
With fear and emptiness behind it
With weakness and failure

Addicted....
I shudder at the thought
Red this morning
Brown tonight
Now sleepy calm
Wish I could do without

Looking at others
That used to be me
Trying to recover
Always a wee bit out of reach
Putting off my envy
Putting on my mask
Feeling like a stranger to myself

Trying to discover
What matters now
A few steps still to go
Up the spiral

Arlene, Maureen and Margaret

housing on health described in earlier chapters.

Some months later, working with a mother and toddler group who were exploring their feelings about food and feeding young babies, the idea of making a slide/tape was raised again. The members of this group felt unsure as to whether they could do this and so the damp housing presentation was shown at the next meeting, to demonstrate how another group in the area had tackled it. There was a short silence after the slide/tape ended and a number of the women looked faintly embarrassed. Although the women liked hearing it, they felt the the Scots language was not 'right'. An animated discussion followed about why it was not right and what it felt like to have your own language looked down on. In the end this group felt they wanted to make their own presentation in their own language and presented it to different groups of professionals, not only in Edinburgh but at a Glasgow seminar of nurses and health visitors (Who Knows Best? 1986).

Producing Videos

Working creatively to express ideas and views to others involves an active learning process. Members of the Middle House Stress Centre were interested in making a video about their own involvement with the psychiatric services and the meaning this had for them. The local video project workers Barbara Orton and Joel Venet from Pilton Video were in tune with the principle that the members should control

---

Song from the WGAG Campaign

(to the tune of the Jeely Piece Song)

CHORUS

Oh you cannae close the Western
Cos it's very close to us
Several hundred poorly weans
Just cannae take the bus
Its a long way for their mums and dads
To go across the toun
And all nigh im-poss-ible
To go to Livingston

Oh, you cannae close the Western
Cos it's very dear to us
Its saved a lot of tiny lives
The staff are marvellous
You should have done your homework
You should have made your plans
Cutting back this service, shows we're not safe in your hands

Oh, you cannae close the Western
Cos it really isnae fair
There's an awful lot of children
In the north of Edinburgh
You've closed down Leith and Elsies and we've got to draw the line
Hands Off the Western
Or you're no friend of mine.

the whole process of production and editing. In the early stages, group members took copies of each shoot home with them, to look at in the privacy of their own homes, before having to look at them in a larger group. At each stage of the process, they had the last word on what was included. This, again, involved a concentration on people's own words, what they conveyed and what exactly they wished to say and an intense dialogue developed between members of this group. The learning process was valued by the whole team and the video workers spent months patiently working with us on the programme (After You Leave the Surgery 1988).

The effect on the group members who made it was also quite profound. The effect, for example on seeing yourself 'from outside' was quite cathartic. One person felt very moved and encouraged when they saw a shot of themselves walking down the street 'just looking like anybody else' – not like an outsider. The video has been used extensively for training purposes and always produces a strong response as the direct impact of the language, coming out of people's suffering communicates itself to the audience.

The use of more creative means of expression adds another possibility for people to name the world as they see it – and to be more visibly seen by others. It links to ideas about the role of culture and arts in making visible the debates which are taking place in society – and it is also an enjoyable and creative learning process.

Problem-Posing or the 'But why?' Approach

The Freire approach to education is sometimes called the problem-posing method of education. In group discussions or learning circles, people's statements about the world are often turned into questions that need to be explored. Rather than a type of closure which accepts statements as the end of the thinking process, people are encouraged to develop a richer dialogue by seeing statements as the start of a process of mutual exploration. David Werner, who has worked on community health programmes in Africa for many years calls this the 'But-Why method'.

The child has a septic foot
But why?
Because she has stepped on a thorn.
But why?
Because she has no shoes.
But why has she no shoes?
Because her father cannot afford to buy her any.
But why can he not afford to buy her shoes?
Because he is paid very little as a farm labourer
But why is he paid so little? etc etc.

(Werner, D 1982)

Questioning is an active stance to take, rather than a passive acceptance of what is. Sometimes it seemed as though people felt they did not have the right to question prevailing ideas and as workers it was important to try and create a climate where this was seen as acceptable and normal. This approach obviously challenges our own view of the world and how much we, as workers, collude in a type of self-censorship of important issues or a reluctance to challenge orthodoxy.

Often when people talked about their lives and concerns, they were aware of contradictions which stopped them moving forward and on a personal level these were sometimes quite hard to voice. The women looking at depression around childbirth had been aware individually that their own experience was not fully consistent with medical explanations of this 'illness' but it was not until they started to feel safe in each others company that they got in touch with this internal understanding and began to share these views.

This confusion or dissonance seems to fall into the realm of 'uneasiness or anxiety' as portrayed by C Wright Mills (1959) in his argument for the development of the 'sociological imagination' – a quality of mind which makes the links between 'the personal troubles of milieu' and the 'public issues of social structure'. He suggests that in order to formulate issues and troubles we must ask what values are cherished yet threatened and what values are cherished and supported? He suggests that people experience 'well-being' when their cherished set of values or ideas are not under any threat. When they cherish values but do feel them to be threatened, they experience a crisis – either as a personal trouble or as a public issue. If, however, they are unaware of these cherished values, but still aware of a threat to them, they experience a sense of 'uneasiness' of anxiety. This unawareness comes about because their private troubles have not been widely formulated or understood. If your own experience is not expressed elsewhere – in the media or through language or by discussions with health professionals – does it exist in this silence?

This aspect of oppression has also been noted by those writing about the development of feminist consciousness in the 1970's,

'we can only grasp silence in the moment in which it is breaking. The sound of silence breaking makes us understand what we could not hear before. But the fact that we could not hear does not prove that no pain existed'.

(Rowbotham 1973)

This form of collective sharing of experience, critically re-examining popular assumptions has a direct link back to the consciousness raising groups that were a central part of the women's movement in the early 1970's. The women's health movement which arose from it had a direct influence on many of the early community health projects and this collective approach to re-examining dominant ideas which do not fit with your experience. The 'but why' stance seemed to create an atmosphere which allowed people to explore areas which had been hitherto 'forbidden'. By this, I mean that either they had not felt they had the right to question certain things or that their own sense of 'uneasiness' had not been formulated or understood more widely.

A discussion group in the Middle House Stress Centre were informally discussing their experiences of being in psychiatric hospital as in-patients. The issue of labelling came up – how some people were labelled as psychotic or neurotic. After a short silence, one member suddenly said 'when I was in hospital the second time I didn't tell them about my voices.' There was a slight hesitation and another period of silence and then one by one, a number of other people also confirmed that they too had hidden their experience of hearing voices. This was because they knew that if they were to be diagnosed as psychotic, the treatment was likely to involve the use of major tranquillisers, which had strong side effects they disliked and made them feel doped or even their removal into a different secure ward.

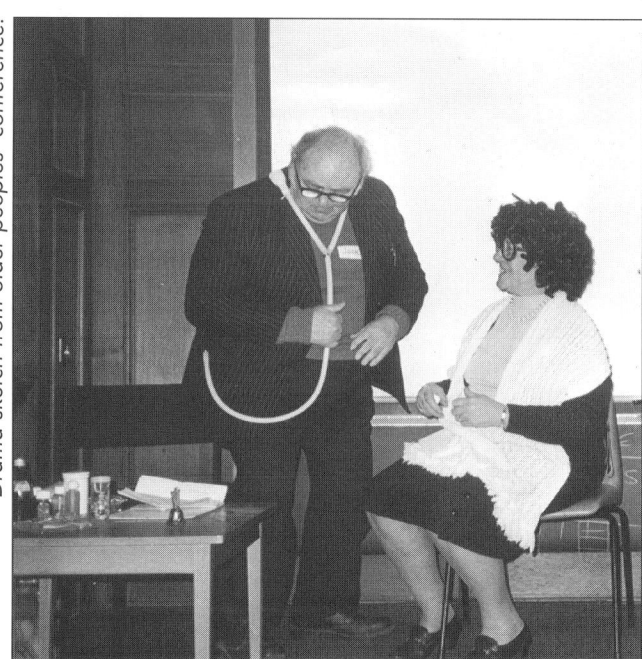

Drama sketch from older peoples' conference.

There was a lot of laughter as the discussion progressed, as though it was a relief to be able to share this very private view with others who understood. Most of the members had not expressed this before to anyone. They also shared aspects of this experience – how they understood it and coped with it. For some it had been terrifying, for others it was not so bad. For most people it had ceased as they got better. 'Naming' their experience in the company of others, was the beginning of developing a different understanding of what it might mean in relation to the dominant view of 'madness'. It reduced a lot of fear and anxiety and led to further discussions which critically examined the labelling of mental illness.

Over recent years, the whole issue about people hearing voices has been given much more prominence. There have been a number of conferences, self-help groups and TV documentaries challenging the view that the existence of voices in your mind should always be viewed as a psychotic occurrence. This example outlined above took place in 1988 before this more public debate began and can be seen as an indication that there is probably a much larger, rich resource of 'private' accounts of health that are often untapped and unused in developing an understanding of our emotional and physical health.

Action/Reflection

The process of digging down to expose the root causes of problems can be very difficult as they might seem intractable and overwhelming. In the above story of the child with the septic foot, for example, the root cause would probably lead to an analysis of poverty and inequity in society. C, Wright Mills recognised that this understanding of the larger historical context in terms of its meaning for individuals had a dual nature – 'in many ways it is a terrible lesson; in many ways a magnificent one'.

An appreciation of broader societal influences can be depressing if we want to feel we are trying to change things. While in dreams we might sometimes wish to change the world overnight, most workers want to be able to engage in meaningful and purposeful activity in the cold light of day on a wet Monday morning.

The Freirian concept of 'praxis' or action/reflection encourages an active stance to these problems and prevents us merely indulging in verbalism – talking endlessly without action, or action for action's sake, without thinking what we are doing. Kirkwood defines the idea of praxis as,

'action preceded, accompanied and followed by reflection, and/or reflection with ongoing commitment to action.'

Campaign Lessons

The campaign to retain services at the local general hospital started in December 1988 when a rumour that the children's wards were to close was confirmed. Strong local protest, and the intervention of the Secretary of State helped to keep the wards open and the Western General Action Group celebrated its success. The following year, the Health Board announced a £22 million shortfall and outlined a plan for major cuts throughout the region. This included plans to close the children's wards, the maternity unit and the childrens and adults A&E Department. The campaign quickly re-formed and eventually won their demands in 1994, after a six year campaign. It was a long, persistent and successful community campaign with many ups and downs, providing a wealth of stories and experiences about the struggle for citizen participation.

The particular aspects which will be drawn out in this section show how the process of action/reflection helped the group to become more consciously aware of their own learning that had taken place through the action they had been involved in. This also helped in the development of campaign strategies.

At a review of its work in April 1991, the WGAG took time to reflect on what they had done so far and the different tactics they had employed. This assessment and analysis of the various strategies that had employed led us to begin to see why some were more effective than others, what areas had been neglected, what needed to be done and what 'input' was needed or what did we need to know more about.

Working with an artist Mary McCann the group were able to construct in a visual fashion, the ups and downs and the stages in the campaign which they saw as a snakes and ladders game and this was eventually produced as the poster called 'Doctors, Decisions and Democracy'. The action the WGAG had undertaken at different times had been based on certain assumptions. As these were tested out, new strategies developed.

Assumption 1. The rightness of the cause. Mass protest will make them change their minds.

This was the initial response by the community and the WGAG. They were so outraged that the Board was even thinking of closing this local facility that they felt right was on their side and that if the Board saw their anger and understood their concern, they would change their mind. This involved them holding large, well attended public meetings, and demonstrations at the Health Board headquarters.

Lesson 1. They realised with some disbelief, that the Board could ignore protest if it wanted to – it was not accountable to anyone except the Secretary of State.

Assumption 2. There is a logical solution. If a reasoned case is presented, they will listen.

As a result of the failure of the first tactic, the WGAG next tried to understand why the Board was even thinking of closure. On what basis were they making this decision? Confusingly, despite their financial crisis they kept insisting that money was not the main problem – the A&E Department was 'not safe' and could not provide the level of care that was needed. The WGAG then began to look into the different reasons put forward for closure, examined the Health Board's own research and met with public health doctors and other professionals who were familiar with the issues. This became even more confusing. The WGAG realised the Health Board was not making a rational or logical decision. It even rejected its own research because it did not support the decision it wanted.

Lesson 2. This led the group to realise that the Board did not seem to be taking a logical decision but a political decision and it was being influenced by other strong pressures.

Assumption 3. If we find out who is influencing the Board, we might have more impact.

The group then began to look into how the decisions were made and to make more contact with individual Board members to try and understand how the process worked. It was quickly apparent that the Board was very heavily dependent on the opinion of the area medical committees of GP's and hospital doctors. It is common knowledge that medics often indulge in 'shroud waving' – suggesting that there will be dire consequences and that people will die, if Health Boards do not follow their advice. This was an argument used a number of times in the campaign. Whether or not there might be some truth in the argument was not up for public discussion, only doctors knew the facts!

Individual consultants could wield a lot of power and 'speak for' medical opinion. This was often very much an individual opinion and was more a reflection of local medical politics and empire building than the considered opinion of the whole profession. This outraged the WGAG who wondered how a small handful of people could decide to remove a service which affected the lives of so many thousands of people. The people who were exerting this influence were also hidden from public scrutiny. It was very hard for the group to find out who sat on these committees. They were invisible and unaccountable.

The other powerful influence was that of the executive members of the Board. As 'insiders' they were privy to a great deal of information and operated the communication channels to the area medical committees and other professional interests. They could imply that things could or could not be done or that the costs would be too high. The non-executive members of the Board did not have the same information at their fingertips and a number of them expressed their frustration with this state of affairs. In an evaluation of the experience of being involved in the campaign, members were asked what they had learnt by working in the campaign. One member wrote, in terms of the way the Health Board works,

'That the Health Board can be quite difficult to get at as the goal post seemed to change over the length of the campaign. We thought that the Board was influenced by the Chief Medical Officer and by the General Manager but this did not always seem to be the case. Doctors, nurses, GP's committees and other sources have a bearing on how they work. I don't think the Health Board members really have that much of a say in what goes on, I think they do more or less as they're told.'

Lesson 3. The group began to understand that power was wielded by a number of different groups who were unaccountable and invisible. The public health board meetings did not reveal this and lay people had little say in the whole process.

Assumption 4: Using the democratic structures we do have, might influence events.

In the months leading up to the 1992 General Election the WGAG ensured through a vigorous lobbying of all party candidates that the closure of the casualty department at the Western became an election issue. A local marginal seat had its effect on the political debates and all candidates supported the WGAG enthusiastically and promised to do their utmost to ensure that the casualty dept. was brought back to the area. Finally the Secretary of State, Michael Forsyth intervened and instructed the NHS Executive in Scotland to ask the local Health Board to review their decision about A&E services and in particular review the service at the Western General hospital. The group was encouraged but sceptical and the feeling was 'just because there's going to be an election, they're going to pretend to listen to us'. However, the penny then dropped – because of the vote, they had to listen to people and maybe this should be translated into local health politics.

Lesson 4. If Health Boards or purchasing teams were accountable, and come under some form of democratic control, it would enable the community to have more leverage over decisions which affected their lives.

This understanding of how the health service structure limits community involvement was a key aspect for the core members of the campaign. Their experience and analysis of power and control in the health service is backed up by many academics and researchers in the health field.

Judy Allsop, writing about health policy in the 1980's came to the conclusion that there were two major factors which hindered the democratic process in health care in Britain and made the NHS resistant to change.

'the two major factors responsible are the power of the medical profession as decision-takers in the service and the operation of the NHS itself....at the level where policy is implemented, at the local level in the health authorities, members and chairmen appear from the research studies to be relatively impotent in

CHAPTER 7

Doctors, Decisions & Democracy ~
Campaign lessons from the Western General Action Group, Edinburgh, 1989-93

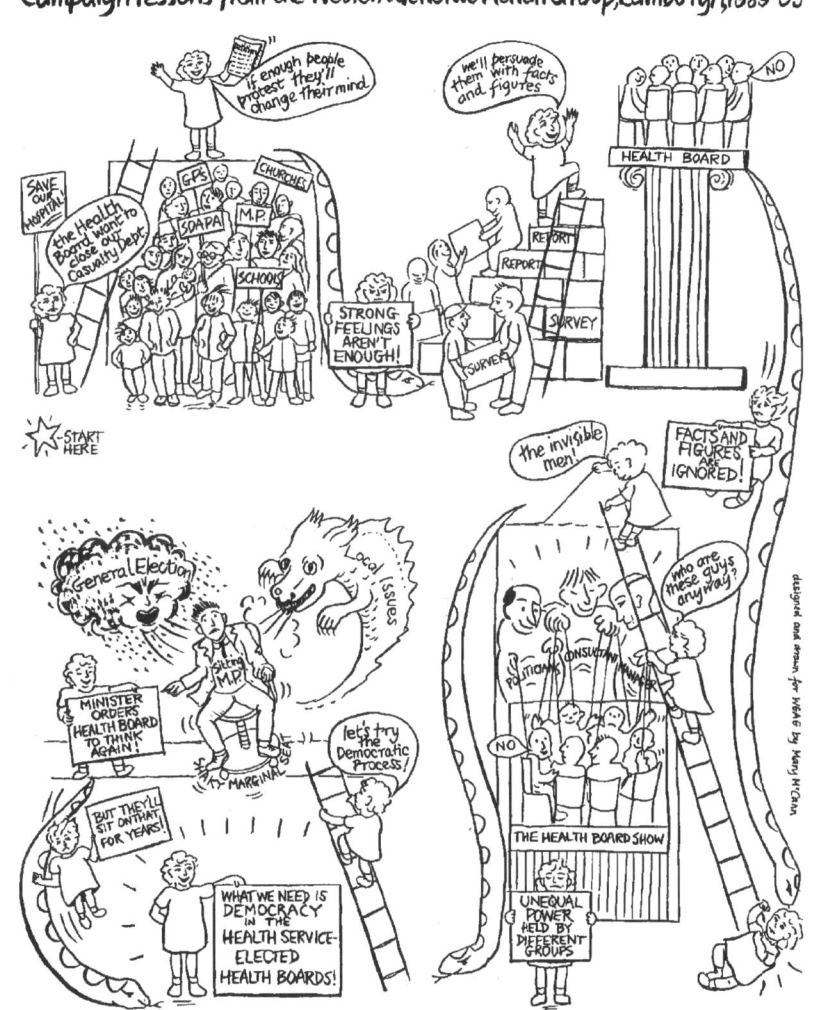

The Western General Action Group has campaigned to keep Accident and Emergency Services, and other services, at the Western General Hospital, for the people of North Edinburgh. A book with full history of the campaign is available from: WGAG, c/o The Health Hut, 3 West Pilton Park, Edinburgh. Tel. 031 332 0871.

123

making policy decisions which go against the interests of service providers, professionals or administrators, even if they wish to do so. Unlike local authorities, health authorities lack legitimacy. They have not been elected and evidence suggests that there is uncertainty about whom or what they represent.'

Although the health service has changed enormously since the 1990 Reforms, these observations still hold true. She extends this comparison with local authorities in terms of the relationships between professional and administrative staff and the link with the community interest.

'there is no necessity for members of a health authority to sharpen their minds in preparing a local health policy for their area as they do not have to face an electorate. This means that knowledge of health services and issues in health are in general low, even among the politically aware....professionals continue to dominate both conceptions of health and resource allocation within the service... and health authority members are largely irrelevant to the actual running of the service.'

(Allsop, 1984)

Allsop's comment on the lack of public knowledge of the health services and health issues can only be countered by grappling with it, learning about it, re-defining it when necessary and drawing more people into that process. There is value in knowing why you feel powerless, rather than just feeling powerless and this knowledge and awareness, coming out of the action/reflection process, can open up possibilities for change.

Through their action, the WGAG began to get a feel for the way powerful interest groups dominated the agenda and how the public was marginalised in the decision making process. The worker's role was to provide opportunities for reflecting on and analysing this together, as a group, so that this new learning was made more conscious and available – in Freire's terms, this was 'knowing that you know'. However, knowledge is the power to know, to understand but not necessarily the power to do or to change. Knowledge is power only for those who can use it to change their conditions.

Conclusion

The title of this chapter 'We make the road by walking' is taken from the title of a book covering conversations between Paulo Freire and Myles Horton – both pioneers in education for social change. It carries the sense of acting and reflecting on the world and engaging in a concrete process that creates real meaning. The examples presented here attempt to demonstrate the way we adapted some of Freire's key ideas into our everyday practice.

Sometimes it was possible to develop more formally distinct learning programmes or sessions with groups but it was also necessary to be flexible and respect the group's other tasks. For example, in the field of mental health, the main task in the initial stages of some support groups was to help people express themselves and to offer emotional and practical support. Encouraging a safe climate for people to move on and critically examine their experiences could take a lot longer. The worker's role can be seen as listening actively and constantly looking for and creating opportunities for learning – both formal and informal.

Freire's ideas sit comfortably with some of the other major influences on the development of community health initiatives. As mentioned earlier, the women's health movement was centrally concerned with issues of power and the de-mystification of knowledge. It emphasised the importance of collectively sharing ideas and validating personal experience as a starting point in developing new knowledge and that 'naming our bodies' for ourselves was a political act. Naming our world – our bodies, ourselves. There was an emphasis on the importance of learning together collectively and creating new knowledge and challenging dominant definitions which did not match with experience.

'imposing definitions is an exercise of power which mystifies and hinders people's thinking for themselves. Resisting others' definitions by searching for the connotation of words is to insist on the importance of demystifying things and thereby developing political awareness. That awareness is seldom acquired by acting alone.'

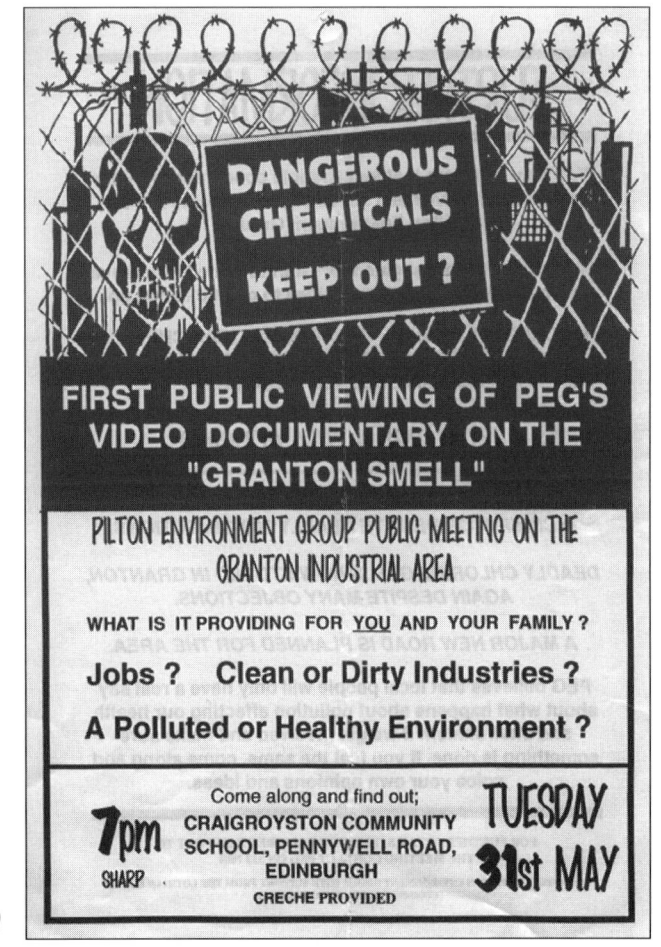

(Rees 1991)

References

Allsop, J (1984)	Social Policy in Modern Britain, Health Policy and the National Health Service Series, pp 226-230. Longman
Arnstein, S (1969)	A Ladder of Citizen Participation, Journal of the American Institute of Planners, 35, 4 July
British Medical Journal (1994)	Increasing inequalities in the health of the nation, BMJ, Vol.309, Editorial, pp 1453-4, 3 December
Edelman, M (1974)	The Political Language of the Helping Professions Politics and Society
Hope, A, Timmel, S and Hodzi, C (1986)	Training for Transformation. Mambo Press
Macdonald, J (1993)	Primary Health Care: Medicine in its Place. Earthscan, London

Paulo Freire

Freire, P (1972)	Pedagogy of the Oppressed. Penguin, Harmondsworth
Freire, P (1985)	The Politics of Education: Culture, Power and Liberation. Macmillan, London
Horton, M and Freire, P (1990)	'We Make the Road by Walking' Conversations on Education and Social Change. Temple University Press, Philadelphia
	Note: The title of the book comes out of the conversation between the two men, where Freire adapts a line from a proverb by the Spanish poet Antonio Machado which reads 'you make the way as you go'.
Rees, S (1991)	Achieving Power, Practice and Policy in Social Welfare. Allen & Unwin
Rowbotham, S (1973)	Women's Consciousness, Man's World. Pelican
Wallerstein, N (1993)	Empowerment and Health; theory and practice of community change, CDJ, Vol.28, No.3
Werner, D (1982)	Helping Health Workers Learn. Hesperian Foundation, Palo Alto
Wright Mills, C (1986)	The Sociological Imagination. Oxford University Press, New York

Pilton Health Project Reports

Beattie, A (1992)	The Pilton Portfolio for Health, Approaches to evaluation in a local community health project
Jones, J (1986)	Royston/Wardieburn Final Report
SHAME Group (1993)	Behind A Painted Smile, A Workshop on Post-natal Depression
Howie, Jones and Purnell (1993)	Who is Listening to Local Voices?

Pilton Elderly Project

Report 1992-5, and Evaluation report 1995	Available from PEP, The Health Hut, 3 West Pilton Park, Edinburgh. Contact: Roberta Blaikie. Tel: 0131 315 2146

Video

After You leave the Surgery (20 minutes)	Available from Pilton Video Project (Tel: 0131 343 1151) and Pilton Health Project

Slide/Tape presentations

Who Knows Best?	The different advice and information given to mothers about feeding and weaning their babies is critically examined by this Craigroyston Mothers and Toddlers Group
Home Sweet Home (also now on video)	The different ways in which poor housing affects the health of families

The Last Word: Local Voices

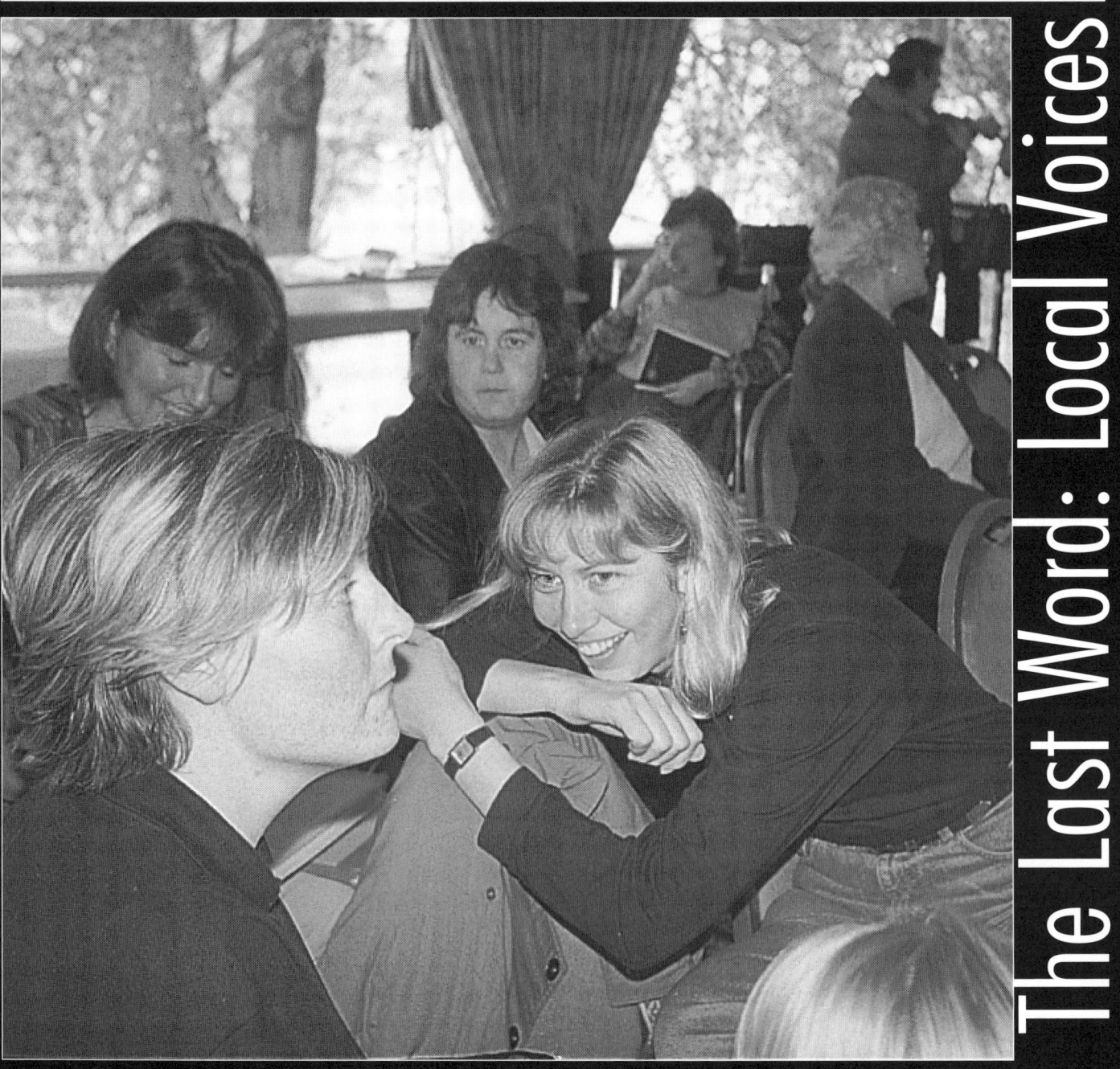

Listening to Local Voices conference.

CHAPTER 8

Introduction

This book has concentrated on the process and practice of community development which is centrally concerned with encouraging people to take more control over those issues which affect their lives. It has also tried to describe the dynamic between different activities and networks. This final chapter looks at how these processes and practices were experienced by local people? It follows the stories of six people who describe their involvement with the project over a number of years and the different issues they became involved with. These personal accounts give a much stronger account of this process including the changes people made as they became involved with different types of activities, at different times and in different capacities. The conversations were tape recorded and are reproduced here with the agreement of those interviewed.

Anne's Story

The Women's Discussion group

In Royston/Wardieburn Centre the health project were running a Women's Health Group and they had a creche which was really good. It was somewhere I could go and take my daughter. It's that hard to get involved in things when you can't go because you've got a wee one. It was just a way to get to know the other women, and to see what they were talking about, so it was a break from the house and somewhere my daughter could actually enjoy as well when she was tiny. I just sort of kept going back and forward there but not sure what I was wanting to do, and I remember one week I went round and there was this girl there and she was saying that she was a having problems with tranquillisers. She had been on them for a good few years and the doctor was trying to get her to come off them. She did want to come off them but she was having a hard time, and she asked if anybody else in the group was on tranquillisers or knew anything about them.

And actually nobody, nobody said anything at all, and I can just remember there was absolute silence. She was actually in tears and I felt terrible for her because I'd been on tranquillisers and I had all the problems with them when I tried to come off them but the reason I never spoke up was because I'd friends in the group and I didn't want them to know. Because at that time, I'm talking about almost ten years ago, there was still a lot of stigma about being on tranquillisers... I wasn't sure what people's reaction would be like. Once before I had mentioned it to a friend – it took a lot of courage to do it – and her reaction was that bad that it made me think twice before doing it again, it was too risky.

But as I said, this girl was in tears and I felt just terrible sitting there knowing that I understood what in a sense she was talking about and I was doing nothing to help. But I waited until the end of the group and people were sort of drifting away, and I went out the door of the centre and I stopped and thought 'Oh Jesus I just can't do this' so I turned and went back in and said yes, I was on tranquillisers and I knew a lot of the problems when I tried to come off them, so I explained the reasons why I hadn't spoken up, that my friends were there and I really didn't want anybody to know. The health project worker said, well obviously you're not the only two people in the area that had been on tranquillisers, I just wonder how vast the problem is. So it really started from there. Actually when I spoke up and said that, about being on them, I felt much better because Jane was non-judgmental about it anyway, and that helps such a lot and the girl just knowing that she wasn't alone and that, you know and plus myself because I hadn't had many people that I could talk to about it either.

The Tranquilliser Group

So from there we decided what would be the next step and we leafleted the whole area and had a phone-in for a whole week. I think it was four of us actually who manned the phones for a week and just said people could phone in any time and talk, you know. We actually didn't get a lot of people, I think about eight but I mean that felt OK and so from there we decided to start running a group in Royston/Wardieburn Community Centre but we were very much working in the dark as well. I was involved in that for about four years.

Housing and Health Group

The other group I was involved with was about housing and health. When I was first married, it was just a very small house and we needed a bigger place so we thought we were lucky to get a council house down at Wardieburn. But later on we found that the house had been empty for about 4 years because of dampness, but I mean we were never told that and didn't realise until we discovered it was dampness and that in the rooms and the kitchen. We complained to the housing department, we got letters and people would come down and say well you've got to keep the house warm, but that was quite difficult because there wasn't any heating at that time in the rooms and we only had a sort of portable heater in the hall, so the rooms weren't getting any warmth. Then I remember someone appearing and saying that they had the answer, *"they say it's condensation and there is nothing we can do because you're no keeping the rooms warm"*.

You're caught in a trap because they were saying you're not keeping the rooms warm and yet there was a lack of space to put a fire in the room, but also the cost of running a fire if there had been space. You just felt caught in a trap and there was nothing – you didn't know what to do. But this person came down and certainly got my hopes built up. She came round and she had a look and she said, *"oh yeah I know what the problem is"*, and I thought great, you know, here's somebody here with the answer and she said, *"you're cooking in the kitchen"*, and I thought what is she talking about. I mean of course I'm cooking in the kitchen – that's what causes a lot of condensation, and I thought she was treating me like an absolute idiot here and I thought she had the answer. I'd built up all my hopes and I was just totally disillusioned. I just shook my head and I mean I just thought this was absolutely ridiculous – treating people like this you know and the kitchen was getting all black with the condensation and I was certainly feeling anxious about the house because of the dampness, and the smell of dampness and you felt bad when you had visitors in, although you tried to keep the house really clean there was always this smell of dampness around.

It actually didn't seem to affect my son but my daughter was prone to a lot of colds and things like that and she ended up getting pneumonia. I mean I was wondering myself if that was the result of the dampness. When she had had lots of cold and things like that I took her up to the doctor and he just dismissed it and said it was just a bit of cold and things like that. But she was getting really sort of stiff necks and things like that and I had to actually help her out of the cot in the morning and she was in sheer agony and you had to sort of help her up and she was all stiffened up and everything. So I went back to the doctor again and I was asked was this my only child and I said no, my son was about ten at the time and I was told I was just being an overprotective mother, which I certainly think I was not. I mean the girl was ill, you had to help her out of the cot, she was really crouched up and that... and actually the doctor came to the house and saw her and after looking back in the records says, we'll get something done about it and asked me if I'd go right away to Leith Hospital and maybe get some X-rays. So they X-rayed her there and said they thought she had pneumonia, so could I take her up to the Sick Children's.

So I trailed all the way up to the Sick Children's which is quite difficult if you've no transport, so we got the bus the way up there and they thoroughly examined her and said yeah, she did have pneumonia but it was the later stages. So I mean they kept her in all day and did tests but they said that it was at the later stages, she was actually over the worst and just to let her go home. I hadn't actually said to them at the hospital or to the doctor that the house was damp or anything like that you know, because I suppose myself I wasn't too healthy at the time.

I didn't relate very much to that until we'd done these photos and slides in the tenants housing and health group. They were talking about problems of the dampness and it was like – yeah we've got the problem as well, knocking our heads against a brick wall because we were all getting these silly excuses that you had as well and so we decided to do something about. We started up an action group thinking, well if a letter doesn't do anything, maybe slides will. So we went round and got slides of dampness in the different houses and that and the overcrowding and we made the slides and then took them up to show some professional people in the university. Although the actual evidence was in front of their eyes, some just really didn't believe us, with these slides they still didn't really believe that people actually lived in houses like that. Then it was suggested that perhaps a survey could be done, a sort of research for the university. They were going to do research on how dampness can affect people's health and that was taken out of our hands. What it was doing was handing over to people who were far more qualified than us to deal with it, and they did a big survey in the local area and I think in their figures it was proved of course that damp is going to affect your health. I think that as ordinary people, they wouldn't really have listened to us but when you had the professional people doing the survey and they actually had figures in front of them, it always seems to be done by figures, then I don't think they could come back and deny it, you know. We got a copy of this survey and what they'd done and I don't know if it was through the survey but they decided later on that they were going to upgrade all the housing, like putting central heating in the house and in the bedrooms and it was just doing the place up a great deal to help people.

The Starting up of the Stress Centre

It was at one of those weekends we were away with the Tranquillisers group, and we were sitting talking and, saying – right, what would have actually be helpful for you at the time, rather than a prescription. We were not saying prescriptions were wrong but not to have them going on for years and years. Some of the ideas that came up through the people that were using the Tranquilliser group was that if only some of them could have just had somebody to talk to, that wouldn't have judged them but just sat there and given them a bit of support, like a listening ear, somebody that had the time... so that's how it came up. It was somewhere you could go and just talk and get a bit of support and encouragement and so basically that's where the Stress Centre started from.

At first I wasn't very sure if I would be able to do that, give other people support, although I had a great understanding but I wasn't sure if I could give a lot of support and that, because I didn't have any group experience or counselling experience or things like that. I got great support and encouragement to be involved in the tranquilliser group, to actually go out and try and do some training that would help me gain some confidence, because although I had the understanding I didn't have the skills to run groups and things like that. I went to Moray House and did some courses out there, I did that for three years. I thoroughly enjoyed that but that was at night time. I didn't go during the day because I still wanted to work with the group during the day, so I went along there and did courses in groupwork and counselling and things like that. At first it certainly wasn't easy – I don't mean the actual work was hard it was just quite difficult sitting in that room and the lack of confidence throughout. You were still trying to gain your confidence but I enjoyed it. I was always thinking – what the heck am I doing here, because other people are far better qualified than I am... but once you actually spoke up then you'd realise that they weren't really, what you had to say was just as important as what they had to say.

So I worked in the Middle House and we started off just on a Tuesday morning there and actually informed the doctors what we were going to do, like all the local doctors and social workers, that we were going to be offering this so if someone maybe went into the surgery, OK they might still get a prescription but it would not be a prescription and, *"OK we'll see you in a month"*, but it could be a prescription and, *"there's a place up the road you can actually go"*, and there will be somebody there that will give you a bit of support. They could actually phone us at home as well, so it wasn't just like a Tuesday, they could phone if they were going through a really bad patch. I've been working ever since in the Stress Centre. It started in the Middle House but we applied to expand and we wanted to offer a Reach Out project. We really felt that people that are needing help deserve more than second best premises and that and maybe we'll have a room here and a room there and we always have to settle for second best. And a lot of that came from members because the PROP Stress Centre is run by members, we're answerable to the members.

I feel this great belief in these people – in the members that are coming to the Stress Centre. Just genuinely caring for them and knowing that their life can get better, than what it is just now. And I know it can happen. At first I was never very sure about how you were going to help this person... I really don't feel that now. I know it can be done, it takes time but it can be done. How do you know you're being successful? You just actually see the change and it doesn't have to be vast, it could just be somebody that's feeling real low and just total disbelief in themselves and in just the gradual change over a few weeks or a few months or whatever. It could be maybe them coming at the beginning and they weren't that bothered about washing their hair, or like just taking care of themselves. An absolute lack of confidence – there's just such a lot of support around, just things like that you know, and as I've said, the members actually run it. I mean they took over and just run it. It's not a management committee now, it's directors and just to see the confidence in them and to know that they've got somebody who actually believes in them and has faith in them, it's such a change. It's just small things, just supporting each other, it's really great.

CHAPTER 8

Marilyn's Story

I first made contact with the health project back in 1985, when my daughter was just months old and I was in a mother and toddler group in Craigroyston Community Centre. I was talking together with the centre worker and Jane from the health project and we began talking about food and children and eventually decided to make a slide tape together, *"Who Knows Best?"*, which was quite exciting. It was good doing it. We got leaflets and looked at them and interviewed Christa who was a health visitor in the area then. We learnt quite a lot together because when I had my eldest girl, whatever the health visitor said – I did it but as time went on I used my own instincts and didn't rely on them keeping me right. When you're a first time mum it's harder. I think you need a lot of reassurance.

We took the slide/tape to a meeting at Strathclyde University. It was mostly health visitors and professionals to do with children. I took my youngest daughter and I was dead nervous, especially as I was on the platform and she was down below having a shot at every seat in the place – I just kept thinking if only she'd keep still! It was my first time ever in speaking to people I didn't know and I felt so nervous I was glad it was over. I didn't think they appreciated it very much this first time – they seemed to think 'who are they, just a group of mothers'. However the second time we did it the audience seemed to listen more.

My sister had five children when she was involved in making the slide tape and she had bottle fed them all. The one thing that was discussed was the feelings she had had when she was in hospital when they put a notice on the baby's cot saying AF or BF. The AF stood for Artificially Fed and the BF for Breast Fed. She felt that artificial wasn't very nice, that it sounded wrong and was quite upset about it. There was a lot of discussion in the group about it. For example one of the mothers was a nurse in the ante-natal clinic and she said that she encouraged all the mothers to breast feed and if they were having problems she'd say, *"oh just persevere etc."*, and yet when she ended up with her first baby she couldn't manage to breast feed and so after that she wasn't so pushy with the other women. There were some older mothers who had not been given any options but to breast feed. I don't know if after all this talk she just thought she'd have a try but my sister then went on to breast feed her next two.

Family Matters

I then went to the Family Matters group in the school. There we discussed how we managed the terrible toddlers and did some play acting! We talked about all different kinds of things – such as how you discuss sex with your teenagers. Because when I was young, my mother wasn't open with us children and I think that was really important that we should be open with ours. I enjoyed that, it was good.

Local Survey

I then got involved with the local survey. To start with there was actually 16 local people and we had training – just to interview each other and see if the questions were right and how long each interview would take. It wasn't a lot of money but it was something in your pocket and the areas I actually did were the areas where I was quite well known and that made the difference.

It was really interesting and I met other women and we carried on those friendships that lasted for years. We actually interviewed 536 families. Once this was over with, a few of us coded all the surveys and did the coding in the school – it was quite easy – and then we went up to the university and fed it all into a computer. Well this was the first time I had ever used a computer so that was another learning experience and I quite liked it. We did the analysis up there. It was getting to know people as well and going out together afterwards. When we interviewed people, they would bring you into their house and show you everything. They were so trusting, were so hospitable and there were some really sad stories. You sort of walk about thinking everything is OK but it's not OK. People were talking about vandalism and unemployment and so on and you just didn't realise how much that it's affecting them. The housing in West Granton (Note 1) for example, is terrible and it's time it was pulled down really – you wouldn't expect any families to live in it. It was so silly how they'd built the scheme. The bottom house was for people with two children or less, the middle for old age pensioners and the top for people with more children.

(Note 1: demolished in 1995)

Women's Health Day

I then helped to organise a Women's Health Day. It involved going round to the local college and asking if there were people who could do sessions and there was the physiotherapist up at the Western that we asked. It was a lovely day and so many women turned up, hundreds came – and it was really good. If you feel you've organised something and at the end of the day it's a failure, then you feel bad but if something's been organised that's well attended and everybody says that they've had such a good day, well – you feel that you've done something worthwhile.

After doing these things I got to know the other women who had young children and all of us had children under nursery age. We used to meet in each other's houses on a Friday, just to have a coffee and a blether and let the kids run about. Because they were under nursery age and they weren't considered 'at risk', there were no places for them. We ended up getting some money to get toys for the Health Project room and did the groundwork in setting up a Childcare Action Group. Our children grew past this age and we got involved in other things but this was picked up later by local women and has developed into the current Childcare Action group (Note 2) which I re-joined.

Then there was a group that the health project and the social worker from the local Family

(Note 2 In 1995 The Pilton Childcare Action group were successful in getting funding from social work and education to set up a childcare centre for local parents who were working)

Services Unit started. It was a very safe group – if there was someone who felt awful, we concentrated on her, so it was important people felt comfortable with their own problems on hold, knowing they would also get some time. After about a year the two workers felt they had put in all they could and after it finished we felt we still needed it and it was suggested that another women and myself should take over as group leaders with them as back up support. It felt quite strange at first because the two workers were the ones who got on with it usually. I used to feel that the others were thinking *"who do they think they are, they used to be like us and now they're leaders?"* They probably didn't think that but you felt that. We had to book the room, see to the tea and coffee and used to take notes and plan sessions. It was a big change. When new members came in it was a bit easier because you were established then. We ran it for quite a long time. It was quite sad to see it finish eventually but sometimes things have to stop and you have to start something new.

Western General Action Group

There was an initial meeting in the health project to explain the rumours that we had heard – that the children's wards in the hospital were to shut. This was at the end of 1988. The classroom was full, there were loads and loads of people there. We started to have meetings every week – we wrote off to the General Manager to invite him to the first public meeting we held and he phoned back saying he wanted to meet us to find out more about the meeting. We went up to meet him and that was honestly the first time I had met someone with that sort of power. He said he could only spare 15 minutes of his time. There was myself and another women from the children's centre and he kept us waiting in the foyer for 10 minutes and we kept saying, if they keep us waiting any longer we'll just have to go – our time is valuable as well. My stomach was churning and it was horrible. Eventually they sent for us and we went in and there were all these big people and they're shaking your hand and saying, *"I'm so and so and I'm so and so"*. Afterwards I thought – what was I worried about – just because he's in a good paid job, he isnae better than me really. He kept asking me why we were having this public meeting and I was being as cagey as him because I didn't want him to know he might have a big fight on their hands. It was important that they didn't find out too much or they might not have come to that first meeting. I realised I had information that he wanted so we were both the same really.

We had very little time to organise because they made the announcement just before the Christmas holidays and we had to have the meeting in the first week of January. I always remember at the planning meetings deciding to have it at the dining hall at the school and thinking we'd give people tea and coffee because it was a winter's night. We then decided against it because we had too much to do but I'm glad we did because there was a good 200-250 people turned up – imagine giving everyone tea and coffee!

It was an amazing meeting. Everyone had something to say and I must admit at the end when I had to give a thank you to everybody I did feel really, really nervous as half the folk in the audience I knew! After that first meeting it was a bit easier when you went to lobby or to present a deputation. Often there was a small group of us and say you had only 2 minutes each to put something across – you had to prepare something beforehand. I learnt to write down a few reminders on cards – just the first few words to get me going.

I was involved with the WGAG for 4 years and the only reason I left was I became employed by the Barri Grubb Good Food Project. It was really quite hard to leave it and every now and again people in the street will say to me – what's happening with the Western? It was hard because I hadn't kept up with what was happening and I'd say, *"I've got another priority now, but I'm not forgetting it"*. A lot of people would say – what are you fighting for, you're not going to win nothing. They've made up their minds, you're wasting your time. Sometimes I'd think they were right, but mostly I'd think sometimes it's better to have a good fight than to sit back and do nothing. I feel that my kids have learnt quite a lot – I mean for four summers they hardly had a summer holiday because they were involved too, but they've got to learn as well, that they can't accept everything as read because there are things you can change. I've learnt not to accept nothing – not to be vicious or anything but just to say, *"look I want to be heard, just like everyone else"*. At the end of the day they might listen or they might not but it's your right for to be open and say your piece.

I've lived in the area for 33 years and as people found out about different bits of the Western closing, they would ring the project or read about it in the paper and stop me in the street. I've even had people at my door saying 'what time is your lobby?' I worked in the local chip shop for 13 years so you're seeing other faces too and can feed back a lot. A lot of people don't read notices and think it's outsiders doing things again.

I've also now been on three different management committees. The Family Service Unit, the Pilton Partnership and the Health Project. On the Pilton Partnership there's a lot of professionals and councillors and private business people but you are treated as an equal. It's amazing how comfortable you could feel. It's hard to explain but when I was younger, they would be called the big shots, you were just the wee ants under their feet, sort of thing, you just did what they told you to do – but now – I'm not saying I wouldn't do what they are saying but I **would** object.

Barri Grubb Good Food Project

It's really good working in Barri Grubb. We now have two other members of staff. When we started it was easier and we had more time but now we're very busy and tied to the minute trying to deliver fruit and veg to four primary schools in the area. There are over 300 children in one school, we take apples and pears and any kind of fruit and sometimes I peel about 100 carrots every morning – the kids love it. We're now at the market about 4 or 5 times a week and get about 10 boxes of apples a week. I found it really quite hard when I started full-time working in Barri

Grubb because I had to give up a lot of these things and let them go gradually. It's hard because you've been there at the start and you want to be there at the end.

It was great in the beginning of the Western Campaign when Michael Forsythe made them stop closing the children's wards and gave us a reprieve. At times it was only a few of us keeping going, a core group but in 5 minutes you're on the phone and it's amazing how many people you can gather. The campaign was a real learning experience. It also gave me confidence to tackle other things because I think if I hadn't got involved with the WGAG I don't think I'd have got involved with the Childcare Action Group again. It was the same sort of fight for something you believed in and I think if I hadn't got involved in the health project in the first place in, *"Who Knows Best?"*, I don't think I'd have been interested in a way, with what else was happening in the community. That was just the first step. Up until then I was just the worker and when I came home from work, came in the house, shut my door and that was it. I wasn't interested in what was going on round about me. Everything just sort of fell into place, nothing really affected me. I was out working, had two kids and everything was fine. When I had to stop work, that's when you realised there was plenty going on around you. It's amazing what you find out, all the different groups there are in the area. I was just interested in my own wee world – you weren't suffering as a person so you weren't thinking of anyone else, sort of thing. You were OK so why worry about the neighbour next door? It's completely different now, I like it, I like being involved.

Robbie's Story

The Women and Food Group in Craigmure School was my first contact with the Health Project. I had been wanting to do something like that, or be part of a group. So I'd asked the head teacher what that project was about and she told me one or two bits and I asked her, you know, would they be interested in this and she said go along and try it and I built up some courage and walked into the community room and asked if there was anything. Christa was the first person I spoke to and it was nice to see a face that I knew because I had met her a few times before when she was a health visitor working at the clinic. I remember asking her... I said I was on lots of different kinds of drugs, food suppressants, you know, stuff like that. I explained to her about the drugs – that I was getting loads of side effects and I wanted to come off them all, so I was needing help with that as well. She said that she would look into it for me and she did. We found out that there were no groups in the area. So we started one.

I got in touch with other women just by talking to friends and people that I'd seen. I didn't really know them but asked them, obviously big women, like myself then, and asked them if they were interested in a group about weight and size and food habits. Wanting to understand why we were overweight.

The first time we met it was in the Community Room in the school. It started off with half a dozen or less, but it soon built up to about fifteen of us. At the first meeting we each explained who we were, our names, a little bit about our backgrounds, if we were married, if we had children. Then we did a questionnaire about how we felt about ourselves. Things like negative and positive lists about ourselves. That's how it opened up. It made us examine our habits, our lives. I think all of us had backgrounds of being really hurt, and had problems.

In the beginning I found it was quite threatening because I couldn't open up, I didn't like speaking to other people, I always felt I was doing something wrong. But slowly you build up some confidence and you tell others. Every time it came round to you to say something I wanted to swallow myself, disappear. There was a lot of crying. And because we were upset it helped other people understand what they were feeling and why.

It went on for months, we closed it after a while because there was a lot of us and every time somebody wanted to come in that was new we had to start at the very beginning, where we weren't at the beginning, we were half way through, we were talking about different things. Eventually there were about fifteen of us.

At that time there was no creche. If there was children came around we had to sort of fit them into a corner and give them a box of toys. But that never worked out – they were always annoying each other and fighting. I think we all took turns looking after the kids but I came to the stage where I couldn't go any further. I had to accept myself. I took turns quite a lot of looking after the children. I think that's about where I started with the creche work.

It started there and I was beginning to get quite interested so I popped along to the nursery in Craigmure school. Went in, met the teachers, played with some of the children once I'd got a wee bit of confidence and I was there, like, three or four times a week. I'd always wanted to look after kids but never had the opportunity. If the parent, you know if they were uptight they always took it out on their kids and I would hear them talking to their kids in a bad way and it made me realise how I was talking to mine. It changed me towards my own children. I started to realise that they had needs as well. But I went through quite a guilt complex about that because I realised for a long, long time my kids must have been through pure hell with me.

Myself, I had lot of work to do because I was on the drugs and I had to come off them. It reawakened in me the abuse I'd had as a child, so I had to work on that as well. I had to start working on that. And then because I was working with the children in the nursery, and I was working on myself, that wakened up something in me that other children were going through and I could spot them out. I could spot the kids that were going through all these troubles and difficulties, whatever. And I wanted to help but didn't know how.

At that time I didn't know what else the health project was about but I obviously knew that there was something good going on and there was a lot of people going in and out the room all the time but I didnae know all that was going on.

Fruit and Veg Co-op

I then started working on the Fruit and Veg Co-op in the school. It was another group that was getting talked about amongst the women and I'd overheard and I wanted to be part of that because a lot of the women, some of the women that were going to the Women and Food group were, like, friends, and they'd started getting involved and I kept thinking 'well if they can do it, I can do it'. Because I thought they were worse off than I was.

I made quite good strong friendships that I've still got, still really friendly with them, because of the Fruit and Veg Co-op. Before that I didn't have any friends. I was in the house all the time. I didn't have any friends. I had come from Morningside but I lived in a hostel then so the only friends I had were the girls that were there. That was before I got married and I got married and came into Pilton. That was a shock! I didn't know Pilton existed! I stayed at home because of, like, circumstances – being beaten up and things like that. I didn't want anybody to see what I looked like. And I was obviously nervous and I had quite a lot of illness as well. I was in and out of hospital and it was very hard just taking the kids to nursery. That was my only contact with the outside people but I wasn't able to talk very much. You know, like I was always wanting to run out the door if anybody approached me.

Working in the fruit and veg was quite good fun. I mean we had to decide what we were buying and what was best buys and you got to know different people. But I think it fell flat on it's face somewhere along the line because we kept running out of money all the time! When it moved along to the Health Hut from the school, I started to get really involved then and I was coming in with a couple of other women that were there and looking after the shop and that felt like my real opening for life. I felt safe and secure and I felt that I could talk to people in there without being shouted down or I was always wrong. And I was beginning to speak my mind. I've never done that before. I was 'Miss Mouse' and disappeared! And with the Fruit and Veg of course there was young mums with young children and the children were always running about, we didn't have a proper playroom.

Creche Worker

I'm not quite sure how I managed to get the job as creche worker but I got it anyway. I seemed to do it all the time, that's possibly why. But we didn't have any proper provisions. The room was empty, there was no carpets. It was like a wee cell, a wee prison cell. No colour. So we got a carpet, and we were starting to buy bits and pieces but I was so fussy it wasn't good enough! I don't know how I came about asking for money, you know like, I needed money and I needed to buy things for the room if I was going to do the job properly and I was given quite a substantial amount of money to buy things. And that was lovely. Because that was like, my choice. I was my own boss and that was wonderful. There was a few arguments with the other helpers about how much you should spend on each item but I decided well, if we were going to buy them we were going to buy something that was worth it and was going to last, so it meant shops like Early Learning. Not everybody agreed with that but I made the decision well if I'm working here, then it has to be **my** decision. I have to have a say in what's going on. So we went out and we bought things and Jane and I decorated it, painted it. Choosing the colour – what colour were we going to paint it. One minute we wanted it really bright and then we were thinking 'no we can't have that, might get the kids too high or something!' So it had to be the really nice, subtle colours. Then we needed shelves, so we got them. Had a special box made for all the other toys.

Well I think I've got the ability to make these children feel safe. It takes time but I've got to make personal promises to them. And one of them is that they'll never be hurt in this room, never, you know like, not smacked. They get little rows but it's safe rows, it's not screamed at. It's nothing to make them frightened. Being told off is just part of life but the way I do it has to be so different and gentle. They get to be themselves in the room as much as possible, whether they're angry or sad or just want to play.

I want to work with children and I believe now that the type of children I want to work with are the really hurting children, that's the ones I want to work with. Because I feel I've got something to give them. Because I know how they feel, been through a lot of what they've been through. The parents of the children, some of the children that I work with were depressed parents, you know, from the baby's birth onwards. And I'm quite jealous of the group they've got because I would have loved to have had that – an understanding when I was going through all that depression. But for me it was like two years of depression, another baby, another two years. I never got any fun out of bringing my children up. I was always frantic.

So that, because I had worked with children who needed a lot of help and I'd managed to do something for them, that gave me a wee bit more confidence, so I wanted to go on from there and do some training. I was so proud when I got my Scotvec through! I couldn't wait to show people 'I've **done** this', you know like, 'I have **done** this!'. I did it at Women and New Directions (WAND) at Craigroyston School and that was another battle. I mean I was so scared. It was OK talking about it and the course went on for four months so you could take your time with it, you know, you weren't rushed too much. I was so scared because I kept thinking 'This isnae for me' or 'I'm going to fail' or 'I'm too stupid to answer questions or have my say' again. But because of the way I was brought up myself, in a children's home, and I'd worked in a children's home and I worked with so many kids, I'd seen so many kids been hurt I've wanted to do something. I kept getting this urge to go on and it was again another challenge. Four months of constant battle, being pushed and even in tears, walking out because I was crying all the time because I kept thinking 'I'm not going to be able to do this'.

I was always being told I was stupid in school because they didn't understand who I was or what I was about. They thought that because I'd been brought up in a kids home I was just somebody with problems. I was treated very

CHAPTER 8

differently from the other kids. I had, you know, little dreams that, you know, I managed to dream of things that I wanted to do and one of them was to be a nurse. When the time came, ...it was the School Leaving Officer then, and he said to me, *"Don't be stupid, you'll never be that, you're not intelligent enough. You'll be fit for washing dishes or getting married and have children"*. And that was my role in life. I wasn't worth anything.

Well, that never left me. It was hard enough when I was younger, constantly being told, and treated badly but when you become a teenager you're so vulnerable to everything and the least wee thing that's said you take on board and it remains there. That was almost the last thing that I could cope with. So I believed him. I believed this person, that I was stupid ... until I got my Scotvec. Oh that was brilliant. I mean, she told me beforehand that I had passed. She didn't have to tell me but I think she knew how scared and worried I was. And even then I didn't believe her, I had to have it in paper, I had to see it for myself, so it's going into a frame to be in the Health Hut. And I've got plans of doing more Scotvec – children with special needs and that.

I did go along to the Keep Fit for Big Women sessions but, again, I wasn't very confident. I could only do so much of it. It's not that I wasn't able, I was just so shy and feeling really bad about myself. But I did do some of it and I did enjoy some of it but there was other parts where she wanted to make you dance, get you to dance and really move yourself and I just couldn't open up like that. So I did go along sometimes. But there was a lot of women enjoyed that. Because most of us were big built, except for the instructress who was built like a skinny wee rake! I was so annoyed, ken like, 'How can it not have been a big woman that was teaching us?' But she was so skinny! She pranced about like this little pixie!

Working in the Health Project, I learned that there are a lot of groups going on and I've met so many people and I know a little bit about the Pilton Elderly Project. I feel like it's not just group of people shut in that room. Like, we're quite good friends and I like to see the old people coming in. I call their bus the 'Granny Bus' cause that's what it minds me of, just a load of wee grannies coming in... Like they'll pop their heads round the corner and say 'hi', I think they just enjoy coming in to see the kids in the playroom.

I wrote a piece for the Annual Report and I was very nervous but I liked having my say and it felt good. You know, when I opened up this book and I was part of it. I don't know so much about the photograph! But I'm changing, I can allow my photograph to be taken. That took time. I didn't feel very important to begin with because I didn't seem to have much of a say except for the playroom. Beginning to say that it wasn't easy along our end, running the creche and I didn't like being forgotten about, that we had problems to deal with – that started us meeting once a month to talk about problems or issues in the creche and that really helped. But like, working in the health project, I started asking more questions and being very much part of, you know, meetings that were going on and having my say.

Jimmy's Story

I came to Edinburgh in 1990. I'd been in a psychiatric hospital in Lancaster for about 5 or 6 years, maybe longer and I was in the short term bit for the last year. Edinburgh Association for Mental Health had found me some accommodation and so I came out of hospital. The front door in the long stay part of the hospital was taboo, if you went near the door you got a doing. Any doors you saw, and folk told you to go out, you didn't go out because the doors always triggered a reaction – if you go near the door, you've had it. So it took about 8 weeks to get me to the front door. The doctor who helped me get out of that place, used to take me for a few steps at a time along the corridor, then opened the door and I went out.

The long stay was like a hospital within a hospital. If you go into most hospitals it looks alright but no many people actually get to the core of the place – it's completely different. Different staff, mostly male and they all wore white coats. Most of them had come from the army or prison service and they had keys the same as prison officers. Their job was to keep you locked up and in line. I think there were about 20 people in my ward – just beds, no privacy anywhere. Nothing for personal stuff – just the bed. Then there was an open bit supposed to be for sitting but you'd be lucky if there were 2 or 3 chairs and just an open space where you walked around. Much the same idea as a prison really although things have changed a bit now.

They used to experiment with drugs. If you asked them what they would do for you, they couldn't tell me. They just kept pumping them into me and ECT as well. I used to shake like a leaf and slaver at the mouth – didn't know whether I was coming or going. I still have bad pain from my kidney. The other one was damaged when I was in the hospital due to a cocktail of drugs and they had to operate and remove it. My remaining one is also damaged and my liver.

When I first got out I realised I had lost a part of my life. The first time I got on a bus I tried to get on the wrong end because all the buses I had known, you just jumped on the back – so I nearly landed on the ground! I also once sat in a cafe for ages waiting for someone to serve me and then I complained and they said it was self-service. I thought, *"what the hell's self-service!"*. It was such a shock that it had all changed.

Through EAMH I was found a flat. You had the security and the freedom to do your own thing. I used to start at one end of Princes St. with all the homeless folk and by the time I got to the other end I had no money left – I couldn't see people with nothing.

Part of the treatment was I had to have some sort of support in the community and I was told about the Stress Centre – it had good vibes with all sorts of organisations so they decided it was the best place for me to go. I just went up to the Middle House and then Anne and Rab came up to see me. I used to go to the Middle House for about 6 weeks for a new members group and then I came across to the Health Hut. The PROP Stress Centre hadn't been built then. It was all being planned then as to how people wanted it to be.

The Stress Centre was very different from the hospital. In hospital you don't speak to anyone and nobody helps you except for, *"You want to make a basket?"*. No I don't want to make a basket. *"Do you want to make a wee clay pot?"*. No I don't! That was the attitude, so I don't really like those places. I found the Stress Centre very helpful. Everyone was the same as you, everyone had a problem. In the hospital you never really knew other people, it wasn't encouraged. I didn't speak to anybody and I didn't like people near me so I just kept myself to myself.

The Stress Centre really opened it out a bit – with talking and so on. Then you come to a point when you feel that the Stress Centre's taken it as far as it can go. You cannae stay in a rut all the time, you have to try and move onto a second stage or you could be in there for the rest of your life. You would just be using it as a club. I can still go back in if I want – I'm still a member so I could just say, *"I'm coming back in for a few weeks because I need some support"*. Workers were there to support you but the members made the decisions. At the end of the day it was members decisions about what we were going to do. It was important otherwise it would have been like another hospital run by professionals. The professionals were there to help you, steer you, advise you, but no really say, *"we're doing this"*. At the end of the day you had the final say.

The happiest time for me was in the Health Hut and in the Middle House which for me gave an atmosphere of professionalism plus I felt they were my friends. I was encouraged to expand my horizons and pushed to achieve my personal goals. If there had not been the Stress Centre here for me I feel I would have ended back in hospital. So in a way that place kept my feet firmly on the ground. I was very aware that my voice did count when workers and members were together making decisions on how the place would run.

Through EAMH I got involved with other projects such as CAPS (Consultation and Advocacy Promotion project) and SUN (Scottish Users Network), became a support worker at the hospital and went to an international conference in Canada. I've also attended MIND conferences here. I've given some of this up but I'm still working with EAMH on drafting a policy for the Social Work Dept. on care in the community.

I next got involved as a volunteer with the Fruit and Veg Co-op when we got money to deliver to elderly people. The we got more funding from the Pilton Partnership for Barri Grubb the Good Food Project. Marylin, the co-ordinator, rang me up and asked me if I'd like to help paint the fruit and veg room and that was it! I've never left since. I wasn't willing to make a commitment to be a worker so I'm a volunteer. I can drop out anytime I like, so I quite enjoy it. I like going to the primary schools. Have you seen 200 school bairns come running at you, screaming and everything! We take the van into the playground and sell out of the back of the van, bairns running all over the place. They buy apples, oranges, and bananas.

Of course everyone says – yes people should be in the community not the hospital – but not next to me! It used to be bad up by where I stay. Kids shouting 'loonies' and bawling at people but you just have to ignore them. Basically, the public should realise that mental illness is like breaking your legs – you can get better. But if you say you've had a breakdown or something, people back off – think there's something wrong. If I'd broken my legs, everyone would be running after you giving you all the help you wanted but with mental illness, you don't see nobody, they all disappear.

Karen's Story

My first contact with the Health Project was when I went to my doctor's, feeling very depressed. By this time it was like – 'you'll have to get me something, I can't tolerate it again, you'll have to help me'. He said he would send me the health visitor. Well she came and said I was to go to the Children's Centre and ask for an application form for childcare and that there was a group for mothers who were feeling depressed and would I be interested? I said, aye, anything as long as it helps, I'll try anything. She must have given my name to Christa and she offered to come along and pick me up to take me to the group. I was desperate to get out and also quite anxious. When Christa came along she was very helpful and relaxed and I really began to look forward to it. I went along myself to Craigroyston Clinic and there was a creche. I must have had the three of them in the creche then. My first feelings were that there was already a group and they weren't very nice to me but it wasn't really that, as I learnt later. People were uncomfortable with no dealing with the important things at that time, because there was somebody new there again. We were able to clear it up after a few weeks.

I remember coming to the Health Hut one time, for lunch and thinking, *"I'm going, I'm going, I'm not staying, I'm going off my head"*. I thought I'd go into the Children's Centre, next door, for an application form and the woman there said – 'oh it's not as easy as that' and I'm standing there with a big double buggy and couldnae get it through the door and I said 'well I'm sorry but I was told by my health visitor to come. *"Oh well you'll just have to wait there the now, until you see so and so"*. So I'm waiting on this woman and she comes and says, *"you'll need to get a visitor to your house, it'll be a social worker"*. I said but I've been sent here but she says it's not as easy as that, you don't just come in and get an application form, there'll be two social workers coming to your house. I mean I was so stressed and angry and anxious.

Anyway two of them came to the house and it was dead funny. There was a bairn sitting in the hall and she said 'oh hello' and then she turned her head and there was me sitting with another one in the kitchen and as she walked through, there was another bairn in the living room – and she says 'is there any more?!'

It was suggested that the group move from the clinic to the Health Hut. Everyone started complaining about the creche and at that time there was no smoking. It was awfully clinical up there, like you were going to the doctors. It was a relaxed atmosphere in the Health Hut, some members liked the clinic and some didnae but it was a group decision to move and we all felt we would be quite happy meeting in the Health Hut.

The first group was for 10 weeks and then you had the chance to say if you'd like to leave or carry on, so we always did that. It was about a year after that that we had the first workshop with the professionals.

I did some training about relationships and ourselves and then another member and I began to run a new group. We did some home visiting for new people. It was really nerve wracking and disappointing sometimes when people weren't in. I mean, it was like – this has taken all this energy, I've come down that road, put the bairns in the creche away along there – and they're no in! It was such a let down sometimes.

I think the first meeting of the group we organised, no one turned up and then one lassie came and she was really nice but she moved again after a few weeks. It was hard to get started but we did eventually and did the 10 weeks and it was brilliant. One woman had come to the first group but had found it too big and she couldn't cope with it, so she came back and it was really good she could come again. I ran the group for nearly 3 years and as a worker it was really good and I enjoyed it. I did more training – 2 courses at Moray House on the SESTA course and I did the ACT training last year, the community work one and I also did groupwork skills training and a four day course on counselling and assertiveness.

Other things I couldn't do because with three bairns, it was a question of time. At one time when one was at nursery in the morning and one in the afternoon and one at school, so I was up and down about 8 times a day! So at these other meetings, you felt you had just got there and you had to go away.

I joined in some of the other activities in the Health Project – I went to some of the Western General Action Group events. It also gave me the confidence to go for my job in the Sitter Service. There were 220 applicants for that job and only two of us were employed. It was such an ego boost, it was great. I've been there three years now.

Sandra's Story

It was about 7 years ago I first made contact with the Health Project, through the Western General Action Group. I was working in the records department in Western and I knew they were going to close the paediatric wards because the girls in the clinic had been told they were moving the clinic to St. John's in Livingston because they were closing the A&E Dept. to children. They were talking about it because they were worried about their jobs. I felt angry about it because of how it would affect my children. I don't have transport and how was I going to get across town if anything happened. In the papers, the Board denied they were doing this and I felt the injustice of that, that they were not being straight, and that it was like the big machine saying no and you knew it was going to affect lots of people and that they had a right to know.

I saw in the paper that there was going to be a meeting and I wanted to go. I put it off for a bit because I was worried how my employers would view me speaking up because I knew I was going to have to say what I knew was the truth, even if the Board were denying it in the meeting. I took annual leave and decided to go, but I took my daughter with me – for moral support! It was a big meeting – I remember seeing all those folk and wondering if I would be able to do it. The adrenaline was going and it was one of the doctors said something which got me going. Then I stood up and said I knew for a fact that the girls in medical records had been told they were going to be moved.

I signed the petition and a list asking people to join the campaign, (the WGAG) but I didn't do anything for a while because my son was just over a year old and I didn't realise I could have taken him to the campaign meetings. I think the next thing was, because I was getting the minutes of meetings, I saw there was going to be a rally outside the health board so I went up and joined in. I didn't really feel part of it but I still wanted to support it. The wards stayed open as a result of the campaign at this stage and the campaign went quiet until almost another year.

I then heard from the WGAG that because of the Board's financial crisis, they were going to make more cuts, including the whole A&E Department. My son had just started nursery by this time so I went along to my first WGAG meeting at the Health Hut and found out I'd come on the wrong day! I felt so stupid but Christa was there and she was really good and helpful and reassured me and told me when the next meeting would be. If she hadn't been so nice I probably wouldn't have gone back. I also got some petitions on that day and took them along to the nursery. I asked if they would give them out. Another woman, Alex asked about it and we both went to the next meeting and she also became a keen member of the group. We both felt the injustice of it very strongly. There was also another mother from the nursery whose child had a life threatening condition and she joined because of that reason.

I started coming to the meetings regularly. At that time I think I was quite naive. I still thought that health was outside party politics – I thought that whatever party was in, they would preserve the NHS because it was different from other political issues. Once you got involved I saw things differently. It was the way the health board treated it. I honestly thought that they would see the injustice of it and that once they saw that they would resolve the issue. It didn't make any kind of sense what they were doing. Even with their deficit, I thought central government would find it somehow. I think we were all a bit naive and the board was very patronising to us.

It was a very busy year and we all had to take on things. I began to take more part because we all had to take turn at speaking at meetings. The first one I spoke at was one called by the labour party in Leith Community Centre. I took my mum and dad and my sister along – if I was going, they were going. They didn't have an option! I remember one of the points we made at the meeting was how many traffic lights you would have to go through to cross the town to the Sick Children's Hospital in the centre. We had worked this out at the last meeting. I'd never met Malcolm Chisholm before – he was chairing the meeting. (He became very involved with the WGAG and later became our local MP). I remember I had to contradict my own unit manager at the time because he was on the same platform. I was feeling like death but I felt the audience was with me.

It was a baptism by fire but I gradually did more and more as we all had to pull together. I also had to go to the City Chambers for a big meeting with MP's and so on. They had asked for a speaker and afterwards asked if I would go onto the Lothian Convention for Health as a representative of WGAG. I joined the steering group and became the Chair of the Convention.

I remember one critical meeting of the health board when they were going to make the decision to close the A&E. It was at a local hospital and all the media and TV were there – there were more of them than the WGAG! The health board started the meeting at 9am and asked us to wait outside. We had asked for a deputation for the main part of the meeting which was supposed to start at 10am. We were left waiting for hours. The secretary kept coming out and telling them there were some problems and it was going to be delayed. Eventually it got to lunchtime and they still hadn't opened the meeting. One of the board members came out for a smoke and I remember telling him we had medical opinion on our side as well and this seemed to change his mind. They eventually let us in after lunch and there were TV cameras and they decided to have a 2 week extension, in order to take further evidence. We carried on fighting and it was another two years before they actually managed to close it.

We began to realise that individual board members felt differently and they didn't all act as one. We began to talk to them individually and invited them to our meetings. I had a phone and so I could do more in that way.

We went to lots of board meetings. We were just supposed to sit and listen but it sometimes seemed farcical the way they were running the meeting. We saw them change their minds with no hard facts to back it up. At one public meeting when they were just about to make the decision again about closure, we began to interrupt and make our points. The Dean of the medical faculty said – this is not a public meeting and the board should not be listening to these people. I interrupted then and said I had as much right to speak as the decision affected me. I lived in the area and it affected my children. It was his tone of voice which got me – it inferred that we had no right – to put you down. But we knew the arguments and we knew the history of the issue. They kept asking different people to look at it or report on it who knew nothing so the same arguments would keep being brought up again and again.

That is a powerful thing – to realise you had that authority. It's realising your own worth. You might feel stupid but you feel the injustice of what they're doing so you've got to say your piece. I remember saying to them – I'll never go away – and we didn't! We kept on and on, even when they'd closed it. We learnt a lot of things. We made lots of alliances with masses of other organisations – pensioner groups, mother and toddlers, the churches, all political parties, health council and so on.

We never had positions in the group, we just slotted in. It was the media that wanted the positions. We all took turns at things. When we had to have a position, like secretary or something, it was for other people, not for us. We used everybody's strengths when they were there. Sometimes, people's children were ill or they had to do other things and they just came in and out as they could.

I was asked to go on the Health Project's management committee and at that time I didn't know what else it did or anything about other groups. I didn't know about other parts of the health project because I had just been involved with the campaign. I came to the AGM and there was a video called 'A Touch of Class' about industrial hazards and things. It was about dockers in London getting a disease from asbestos. One doctor at the AGM said that it went on for so long because they didn't know about the connection. I remember saying that when my dad was an apprentice in the shipyards, Robbs, that they used to throw 'snowballs' of the blue asbestos around at each other. The employers said they didn't know but they did and did nothing about it. I wasn't afraid to question the doctor. It was knowing you are equal and you've got a right to speak. I was next elected chair and I didn't quite know what it would be like but we had training days and it helped to get to know the other committee members.

I was totally amazed at what was involved and the whole concept of the project. I was just in the campaign and I hadn't realised how heavily it was involved in different things and touched so many people. I was really pleased to be part of that, it was nice to be involved and I felt very proud. It was a real sense of community.

Appendix

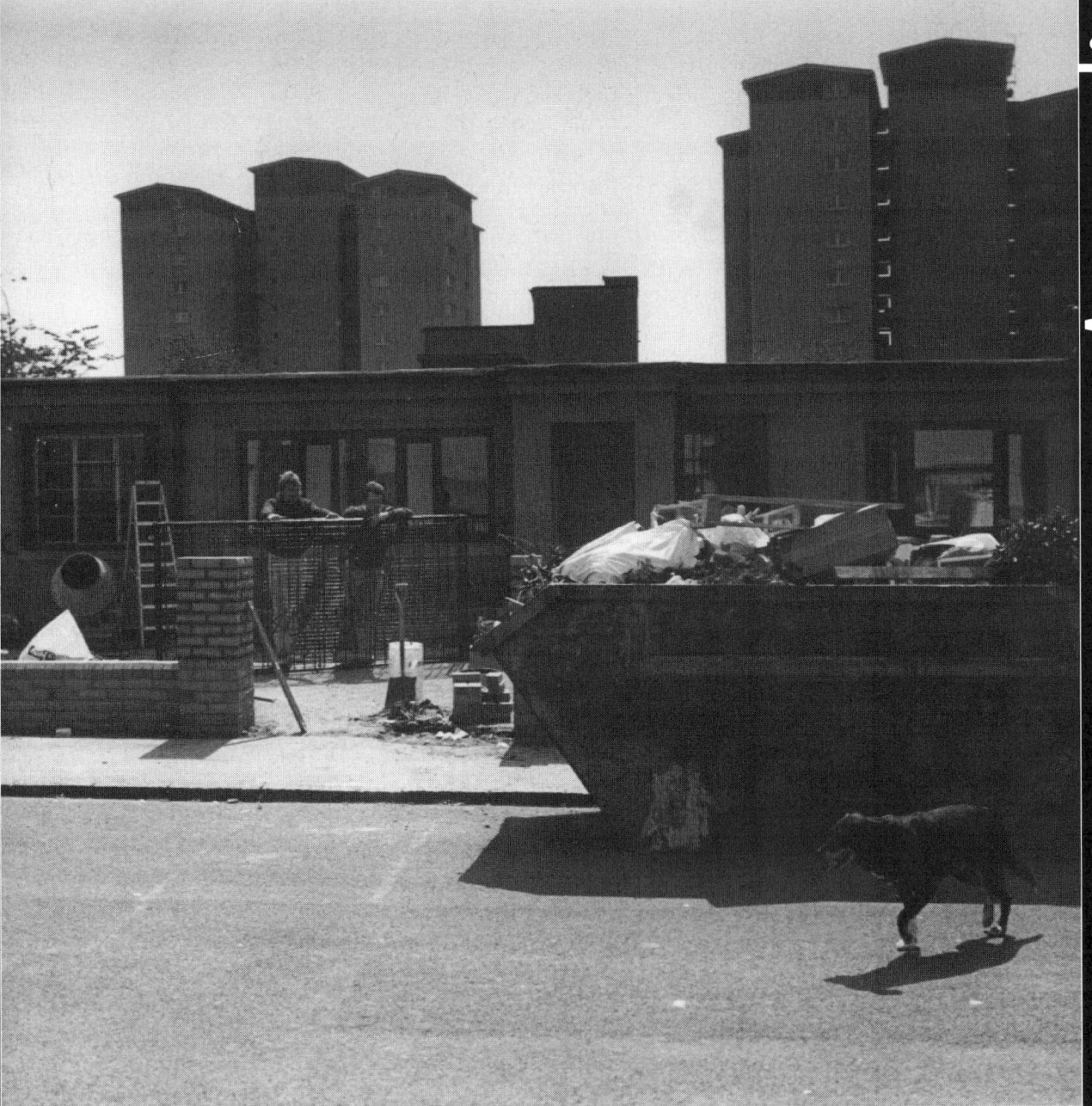

Health Hut improvements and building the Stress Centre next door.

Pilton Health Projects Reports

Minor Tranquillisers, Major Problems. Conference report, Royston/Wardieburn Health Project and Scottish Association for Mental Health (1985)

Tranquillity without Tranquillisers. Booklet produced by Come off it Group (1986)

Royston/Wardieburn Community Health Project. Final report, J. Jones (1986)

Community Development and Health: Developing the practice. J. Jones and C. Wynn-Williams (1986-1988)

West Pilton Clinic Users Group: User participation in practice. K. Alexander and M. Beagley (November 1988)

To be or not to be thin: Women's struggle with food. Conference report, C. Wynn-Williams (1990)

Behind a Painted Smile. Report on a workshop on post-natal depression, Self-Help Around Mum's Experience Group (April 1991)

Keeping Well! 1991 Annual Report, Pilton Community Health Project

We think it's worth it! Survey on women's experience of cervical smears and colposcopy services, Pilton Well Woman Investigation Group and Pilton Community Health Project (1992)

Open University Health and Wellbeing Course. Pilton Community Health Project used as one of the core case studies (1992)

High Rise Living. Report by the Inchcolm Court Flats Group (May 1992)

Pills: Information that's hard to swallow. Study conducted by M. Deans (1993)

Pilton Counselling Service. Evaluation of the first year, M. Bain and J. Jones (1993)

Changes in the NHS: Who is listening to local voices? S. Howie, J. Jones and S. Purnell (1993)

Western General Action Group Reports

Patients' Needs First. W.G.A.G. (1991)

Casualties of Indifference. Report on the effects on patients of the closure of the accident and emergency department at the Western General Hospital, W.G.A.G. (1992)

Emergency Care in North West Edinburgh. Survey of general practitioners prepared by Scottish Health Feedback on behalf of Lothian Convention of Health, Lothian Health Council and W.G.A.G. (1992)